Heart Health~ ~~~~~

50 Low Sodiu~

for Hea~ ~~~~~ ~~~~~

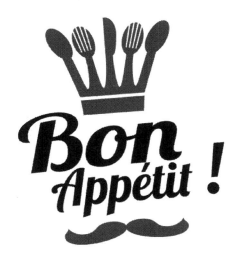

Ann Brown

Table of Contents

Cooking Measurement Conversion Chart

Liquid Measures

1 gal = 4 qt = 8 pt = 16 cups = 128 fl oz
½ gal = 2 qt = 4 pt = 8 cups = 64 fl oz
¼ gal = 1 qt = 2 pt = 4 cups = 32 fl oz
½ qt = 1 pt = 2 cups = 16 fl oz
¼ qt = ½ pt = 1 cup = 8 fl oz

Dry Measures

1 cup = 16 Tbsp = 48 tsp = 250ml
¾ cup = 12 Tbsp = 36 tsp = 175ml
⅔ cup = 10 ⅔ Tbsp = 32 tsp = 150ml
½ cup = 8 Tbsp = 24 tsp = 125ml
⅓ cup = 5 ⅓ Tbsp = 16 tsp = 75ml
¼ cup = 4 Tbsp = 12 tsp = 50ml
⅛ cup = 2 Tbsp = 6 tsp = 30ml
1 Tbsp = 3 tsp = 15ml

Dash or Pinch or Speck = less than ⅛ tsp

Quickies

1 fl oz = 30 ml
1 oz = 28.35 g
1 lb = 16 oz (454 g)
1 kg = 2.2 lb
1 quart = 2 pints

U.S.	Canadian
¼ tsp	1.25 mL
½ tsp	2.5 mL
1 tsp	5 mL
1 Tbl	15 mL
¼ cup	50 mL
⅓ cup	75 mL
½ cup	125 mL
⅔ cup	150 mL
¾ cup	175 mL
1 cup	250 mL
1 quart	1 liter

Recipe Abbreviations

Cup = c or C
Fluid = fl
Gallon = gal
Ounce = oz
Package = pkg
Pint = pt
Pound = lb or #
Quart = qt
Square = sq
Tablespoon = T or Tbl
    or TBSP or TBS
Teaspoon = t or tsp

Fahrenheit (°F) to Celcius (°C)

°C = (°F - 32) x 5/9

Fahrenheit	Celcius
32 °F	0 °C
40 °F	4 °C
140 °F	60 °C
150 °F	65 °C
160 °F	70 °C
225 °F	107 °C
250 °F	121 °C
275 °F	135 °C
300 °F	150 °C
325 °F	165 °C
350 °F	177 °C
375 °F	190 °C
400 °F	205 °C
425 °F	220 °C
450 °F	230 °C
475 °F	245 °C
500 °F	260 °C

OVEN TEMPERATURES

WARMING: 200 °F
VERY SLOW: 250 °F - 275 °F
SLOW: 300 °F - 325 °F
MODERATE: 350 °F - 375 °F
HOT: 400 °F - 425 °F
VERY HOT: 450 °F - 475 °F

*Some measurements were rounded

Introduction

Heart Health is that every American and over the world citizen should be concerned about. Different heart diseases are one of the main death reasons for both men and women. Moreover, cardiovascular diseases often called as "the silent killer" because it cannot be any warning signs before a heart attack strikes.

Fortunately, heart health is under your control. Surely, there're many factors that cannot be changed, such as age or family history, but you can reduce risk of heart attacks choosing a healthy way of life.

Unfortunately, many people do not use healthy habits for various reasons. Some do not have enough time, some do not have enough knowledge, for some people it's too hard. However, you need to understand that your healthy lifestyle is the best protection against heart diseases, so a healthy way of life is the simplest way to live a long happy life.

Properly formulated diet is one of the easiest and most effective ways to reduce heart diseases attacks. Many people do not know what meals to eat in order to keep the heart and blood vessels healthy. That is why I created this book, which contains delicious, easy, and at the same time useful heart healthy recipes for two that will allow you to eat properly, and also reduce the risk of cardiovascular diseases.

10 Heart-Healthy Foods and Nutrients Everybody Should Add to the Diet

1. Avocados - eating an avocado a day may lower your risk of "bad" LDL cholesterol, because these fruits have a rich nutrient profile and don't contain any sodium.

2. Whole Grains - according to a review published in BMJ, eating three or more servings of whole grains a day may reduce your risk of heart disease as much as 22%. The fiber, B vitamins, iron, magnesium, and zinc in whole grains improve your cholesterol and carry oxygen to the blood to lower your risk of heart disease.

3. Beans - beans are packed with protein and heart-healthy nutrients like B vitamins and potassium.

4. Dark Chocolate - you can lower your cholesterol eating sweets. According to a study published in the Journal of the American Heart Association, having 2/3 Tbsp of cocoa with 1/3 cup of almonds each day reduces your LDL cholesterol levels to prevent heart disease.

5. Chia Seeds - a significant reduction in blood pressure for those who consumed the chia flour.

6. Pineapple - according to Medical News Today, one cup of pineapple has more than 100% of your day's vitamin C needs.

7. Cashews - a great source of magnesium, a mineral that may help lower blood pressure.

8. Brussels Sprouts - an excellent source of fiber. The American Heart Association recommends 25 g of fiber a day, and 1 cup of Brussels sprouts has 3.3 g fiber.

9. Peanut Butter - is still one of the best heart-healthy foods. Although the creamy spread is high in fat, it's mostly the unsaturated — or healthy — kind of fat.

10.   Salmon - is a good source of omega-3s fatty acids, which are healthy sources of fat. According to a review published in A Peer-Reviewed Journal for Managed Care and Hospital Formulary Management, two omega-3s, EPA, and DHA, are strongly associated with heart health because they decrease triglyceride levels and help keep blood vessels from clogging.

12 Useful tips to minimize risk of heart healthy diseases

1. Eat heart healthy meals. Make fruit, vegetables, fish, and whole grains the main in your diet.

2. Limit sodium, saturated fats and sweets.

3. Be active. Try to walk at least 10 000 steps per day.

4. Control your blood sugar. Blood glucose should be less than 100 mg/dL

5. Control your cholesterol. Total cholesterol should be less than 200 mg/dL

6. Control your blood pressure. Try to keep your numbers below 120/80 mm Hg

7. Live smoke-free

8. Drink more green tea. It reduces the risk of heart attack.

9. Reach for vitamin D. Nearly 75% of heart patients are deficient in Vitamin D.

10. Have an optimistic outlook.

11. Keep calm. Try to find 30 minutes per day for relaxation techniques such as deep breathing or meditation.

12. More muscle – less fat. Do more physique exercises.

9 foods that help you Burn Fat

Beat your belly fat faster and protect yourself from heart diseases!

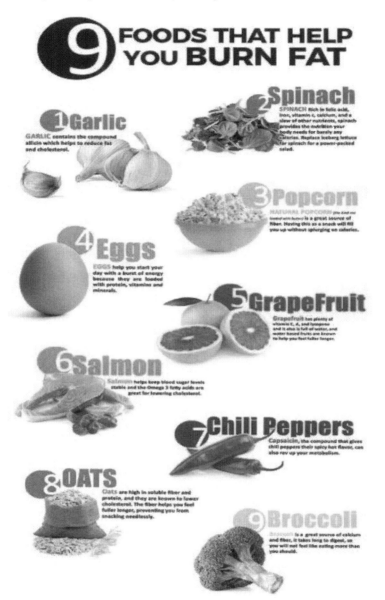

Heart Healthy Main Dishes

Sweet Potato Kale Frittata

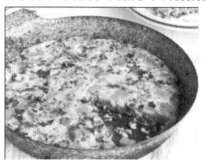

Prep time: 20 minutes, cook time: 10 minutes, servings: 2

Ingredients

- 3 large eggs
- 1/2 cup half-and-half
- 1 tsp salt
- 1/2 tsp freshly ground pepper
- 1 cups sweet potatoes
- 2 tbsp olive oil
- 1 cups firmly packed chopped kale
- 1/2 small onion
- 1 clove garlic, chopped
- 2 oz goat cheese

Directions

1. Preheat oven to 350 F. In a medium-sized bowl whisk together eggs and next 3 ingredients. Set aside.
2. Sauté sweet potatoes in 1 tablespoon hot oil in a 10-inch ovenproof nonstick skillet over medium heat up to 10 minutes or until potatoes are tender and golden; remove and keep warm. Sauté kale with chopped onions and garlic in remaining 1 tablespoon oil 3 to 4 minutes or until kale is wilted and tender; stir in potatoes.
3. Pour egg mixture evenly over vegetables, and cook 3 more minutes. Sprinkle egg mixture with goat cheese.
4. Bake at 350 F 10 to 14 minutes or until set.

Spaghetti Squash and Chickpea Sauté

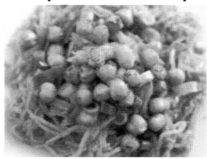

Prep time: 10 minutes, cook time: 20 minutes, servings: 2

Ingredients

- 1 pound spaghetti squash
- 1 small red onion, chopped
- 4 tbsp fresh lemon juice
- 2 tbsp olive oil
- 2 cloves garlic, minced
- 1/2 15-ounce can chickpeas, rinsed
- 1/2 cup freshly chopped parsley
- 2 oz crumbled feta
- Salt and black pepper to taste

Directions

1. Halve spaghetti squash lengthwise with a knife, discard seeds. Place both halves cut side down on a large piece of parchment paper, and microwave on high until just tender, up to 10 minutes. Use a fork to shred squash strands, and transfer to a large bowl.
2. In another mixing bowl, toss onion, lemon juice, and a pinch each salt and pepper.
3. In a nonstick skillet, heat 1 tablespoon olive oil and minced garlic until lightly golden. Add chickpeas and cook for 2 minutes more. Toss with spaghetti squash, 1 tablespoon olive oil, season with salt and pepper. Fold in parsley and onion (and juices). Top with crumbled feta and serve

Nutrition facts per serving

- 245 calories
- 10 g fat (1.5 g saturated)
- 7 g protein
- 340 mg sodium
- 27 g carb
- 8 g fiber

Cumin-Spiced Lamb with Carrot and Radish Salad

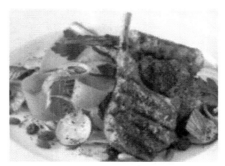

Prep time: 10 minutes, cook time: 20 minutes, servings: 2

Ingredients

- 4 small lamb loin chops (3/4-inch thick), well trimmed
- 3 tbsp olive oil
- 2 tbsp red wine vinegar
- 1/2 tsp honey
- 1 tsp ground cumin
- 1 large carrot
- 3 large radishes
- 1/4 cup fresh mint leaves
- Salt and pepper to taste

Directions

1. In a medium mixing bowl, whisk 2 tablespoons oil, vinegar, honey, 1/4 teaspoon cumin. Also add salt and pepper, to taste and mix well.
2. Heat the remaining tablespoon oil in a large skillet over medium heat. Season the lamb with the remaining teaspoon cumin, salt and pepper. Cook the lamb to desired doneness, 4 to 5 minutes per side for medium-rare.
3. Meanwhile, using a vegetable peeler, shave the carrots into thin strips and very thinly slice the radishes. Add to the dressing and toss to coat. Fold in the mint leaves and serve with the lamb.

Nutrition facts per serving

- 329 calories
- 13 g fat (4 g saturated)

14

- 82 mg cholesterol
- 511 mg sodium
- 27 g protein
- 11 g carbs
- 3 g fiber

Amazing Pork and Vegetable Stir-Fry

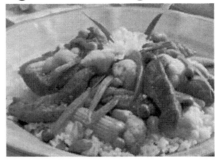

Prep time: 30 minutes, cook time: 30 minutes, servings:2

Ingredients

- 1/2 cup long-grain white rice
- 1/2 pound pork
- 2 tbsp hoisin sauce
- 1 tbsp fresh lime juice
- 2 tbsp canola oil
- 1 medium carrot, sliced
- 1 small red bell pepper, sliced
- A pinch of salt and pepper
- 1/2 cup bean sprouts

Directions

1. Cook the rice according to package directions.
2. In a small mixing bowl, combine hoisin sauce, lime juice and 1 tablespoon water. Mix well and set aside.
3. On a large skillet add 1 tablespoon oil and heat over medium heat. Add the carrots and bell pepper and cook, stirring frequently, until tender, nearly 5 minutes. Transfer to a bowl.
4. Return the skillet to the stove, add another tablespoon of oil. Season the pork with salt and pepper and fry on a skillet, flipping couple times, Pour in the hoisin mixture and cook for 1 minute.
5. Return the vegetables to the skillet, add the bean sprouts (if using) and cook, tossing, until heated through, about 2 minutes. Serve over the rice and enjoy.

Classic Beef & Broccoli

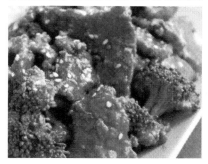

Prep time: 25 minutes, cook time: 25 minutes, servings: 2

Ingredients

- 1/2 pound pork steak, halved lengthwise, then very thinly sliced crosswise
- 1 cup broccoli, cut into small florets
- 2 tbsp low-sodium soy sauce
- 4 tsp rice vinegar
- 2 cloves garlic, minced
- 1 tbsp brown sugar
- 1 tsp grated fresh ginger
- 1 tsp cornstarch
- 1 tbsp canola oil
- 1 small red chili, thinly sliced
- 2 scallions, thinly sliced

Directions

1. In a mixing bowl combine soy sauce and vinegar, add minced garlic. Add the meat and set aside for 5-10 minutes.
2. Place broccoli in a large skillet, add some water and simmer until nearly tender and bright green. Transfer to a plate.
3. Meanwhile, in another bowl mix together sugar, ginger, cornstarch, some soy sauce and vinegar, couple tbsp water.
4. Add the oil to a skillet and heat. Add beef in one layer and cook for 1-2 minutes. Add the sauce and simmer until meat will be tender. Add the broccoli and scallions and toss to combine.
5. Serve with or without rice.

Spaghetti Squash and Chickpea Sauté

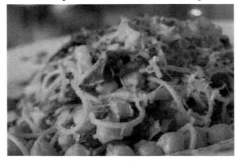

Prep time: 5 minutes, cook time: 15 minutes, servings: 2

Ingredients

- 1 pound spaghetti squash
- 1 small red onion, finely chopped
- 3 tbsp fresh lemon juice
- 2 tbsp olive oil
- 1 garlic clove, minced
- 1/2 can chickpeas, rinsed
- 1/2 cup fresh flat-leaf parsley, chopped
- 2 oz crumbled feta
- Ground black pepper to taste

Directions

1. Prepare spaghetti squash and halve with large knife. Place them on a large paper sheet and microwave on high for 5-7 minutes until tender. Transfer cooked spaghetti to a large bowl.
2. Meanwhile, in a small mixing bowl toss onion, lemon juice and season with salt and pepper.
3. Sprinkle a non-stick skillet with 1 tbsp olive oil and toss minced garlic. Cook until golden brown. Add rinsed chickpeas and cook for couple minutes. Add spaghetti squash and 1 tablespoon olive oil.
4. Top with crumbled feta and serve.

Fusilli with Broccoli Topping

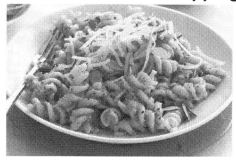

Prep time: 10 minutes. cook time: 15 minutes, servings: 2

Ingredients

- 6 oz. fusilli pasta
- 6 oz. frozen broccoli florets
- 1-2 clove garlic
- 1/4 cup fresh basil leaves or 1 tbsp dried basil
- 3 tbsp. olive oil
- 1 tbsp. grated lemon zest
- Parmesan cheese, grated (if desired)

Directions

1. Cook the pasta according to package directions. Reserve 1/2 cup of the cooking liquid, drain the pasta, and return it to the pot.
2. Meanwhile, in a microwave-safe bowl, combine the broccoli, garlic, and 1/2 cup water. Cover and cook on high, stirring once halfway through, until the broccoli is tender, 5 to 6 minutes. Transfer the mixture (liquid included) to a food processor. Add the basil, oil, zest, and purée until smooth.
3. Toss the pasta with the pesto and 1/4 cup of the reserved liquid. Sprinkle with grated Parmesan cheese if desired.

Spicy Lamb with Veggies

Prep time: 20 minutes, cook time: 20 minutes, servings: 2

Ingredients

- 4 small lamb chops
- 2 medium-sized carrots
- 5 large radishes
- 3 tbsp olive oil
- 2 tbsp red wine vinegar
- 1/2 tsp honey
- 1/2 tsp ground cumin
- A pinch of salt and pepper

Directions

1. In a medium mixing bowl combine oil, vinegar, honey, cumin, season salt and pepper, and whisk to combine well. Set aside.
2. Preheat the skillet over medium-high heat. Sprinkle with tbsp of olive oil. Season the lamb chops with salt and pepper and cook on skillet to desired doneness - 4-6 minutes from each side.
3. While frying, use a vegetable peeler to make thin carrot strips and thin radish slices. Transfer veggies to a large bowl and cover with vinegar mixture. Combine well and serve with cooked lamb chops.

Pork Medallions with Herbs

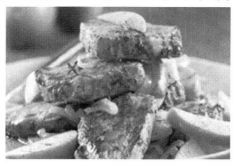

Prep time: 20 minutes, cook time: 30 minutes, servings: 2

Ingredients

- 1 pound pork tenderloin
- 2 medium-sized carrots
- 1/2 pound asparagus
- 2 tbsp olive oil
- 1/2 cup freshly chopped parsley
- 1/2 tsp dried rosemary
- 1 package baby greens and herbs
- A pinch of salt and pepper

Directions

1. In a bowl combine chopped parsley and rosemary. Rub this mixture over the tenderloin and set aside.
2. Boil carrots for 5 minutes, chill. Do the same with asparagus for 3 minutes, until bright green and crisp.
3. Preheat oven to 380 F.
4. Cover the pork tenderloin with salt and pepper, preheat the ovenproof skillet and cook meat for 5-8 minutes until brown. Transfer to an oven and cook until ready and tender.
5. Meanwhile, cut carrots and asparagus into 2-inch-long sticks. Transfer to a large bowl, add baby greens, and remaining parsley. Season with salt and pepper and add remaining tablespoon oil. Add balsamic vinegar and stir to combine. Divide salad among serving plates.
6. Slice pork tenderloin and serve on the top of the salads.

Ravioli with Easy Tomato Sauce

Prep time: 5 minutes, cook time: 15 minutes, servings: 2

Ingredients

- 1 package (16-18 oz) small cheese ravioli
- 1 small clove garlic
- 2 tbsp olive oil
- Salt and pepper
- 1 large tomato, stem removed
- 4 tbsp freshly chopped basil leaves
- Grated Parmesan cheese, for serving

Directions

1. Cook the ravioli according to the package directions.
2. Meanwhile, mince the garlic into a large bowl, then stir in the oil and season with salt and pepper.
3. Cut 1/4 inch off the top of the tomato and finely grate the cut sides into the bowl until you reach the skin; discard the skin. Stir to combine, then fold in the basil.
4. Spoon the sauce over the ravioli and sprinkle with extra basil and Parmesan if desired.

Nutrition facts per serving

- 326 calories
- 11 g fat (2,5 g saturated)
- 28 mg cholesterol
- 354 mg sodium
- 13 g protein
- 46 g carbs
- 3 g fiber

Quick & Easy Chicken, Green Bean, and Bacon Pasta

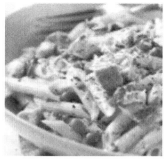

Prep time: 10 minutes, cook time: 25 minutes, servings: 2

Ingredients

- 6 oz penne pasta
- 4 oz green beans, trimmed and halved
- 2 slices bacon
- 1/2 pound chicken breasts, boneless and skinless, cut into 1/2-inch chunks
- 1 tbsp fresh lemon juice
- 1 egg yolk
- 2 tbsp half-and-half
- 3 oz baby spinach
- 1 oz Parmesan cheese, grated
- 2 scallions, sliced

Directions

1. Cook pasta per package directions, adding green beans to the pot during the last minute. Reserve 1/2 cup cooking water; drain, then return pasta and green beans to pot.
2. Meanwhile, in a large skillet on medium-high heat, cook bacon until crisp, nearly 3-4 minutes per side. Transfer to a paper towel and break into pieces when cool. Discard all but 1 tbsp bacon drippings and return pan to medium.
3. Cook chicken until golden brown and cooked through, tossing once, 6 to 8 minutes; remove from heat and toss with lemon juice. In a small bowl, whisk egg yolk and half-and-half. Toss egg mixture with pasta and green beans, then fold in chicken, spinach, Parmesan, and 1/4 cup pasta water, tossing to coat

and adding more pasta water if needed. Fold in scallions and
top with bacon.
4. Serve and enjoy

Nutrition facts per serving

- 570 calories
- 13 g fat (5 g saturated)
- 43 g protein
- 355 mg sodium
- 70 g carb
- 5 g fiber

Heart Healthy Bean Burrito Bowl

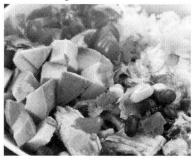

Prep time: 20 minutes, cook time: 25 minutes, servings: 2

Ingredients

- 1 cup cooked brown rice
- 1 small avocado
- 1/2 can black beans
- 2 tbsp fresh lime juice
- 2 tbsp olive oil
- 1/2 tsp. ground cumin
- 1/4 head romaine lettuce
- 1 tbsp dried cilantro
- 5 cherry tomatoes, cut
- 1/2 small red onion
- 2 tbsp low-fat sour cream
- Tortilla chips, lime wedges for dressing
- Hot sauce to taste

Directions

1. In a small mixing bowl, whisk together the lime juice, oil, and cumin.
2. Divide the rice and beans among serving bowls. Top with the lettuce, cilantro, tomatoes, and avocado.
3. Sprinkle with the red onion, then drizzle with the dressing. Serve with sour cream, tortilla chips, lime wedges, and hot sauce, if desired.

Delicious Pineapple and Ham Fried Rice

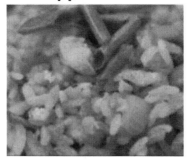

Prep time: 5 minutes, cook time: 30 minutes, servings: 2

Ingredients

- 1/2 cup long-grain white rice
- 1 tbsp olive oil
- 3 oz thick-cut sliced ham
- 1/2 pound pineapple
- 1 small red pepper
- 1 small red onion
- 1 jalapeño
- 1 piece fresh ginger
- 2 clove garlic, minced
- Fresh cilantro, chopped

Directions

1. Firstly, Cook the rice according to package directions.
2. Meanwhile, heat the oil in a large nonstick skillet over medium heat. Add the ham and cook, tossing occasionally, until lightly brown, about 3 minutes. Add the pineapple and cook until beginning to brown around the edges, up to 3 to 4 minutes. Season with salt and pepper and cook for 2 minutes more.
3. Add the onion and cook, tossing, for 3 minutes. Add the jalapeño, ginger, and garlic and cook, tossing occasionally, until the vegetables are just tender, 2 to 3 minutes more.
4. Add the cooked rice to the skillet and toss to combine. Serve with cilantro and enjoy.

Nutrition facts per serving

1. 345 calories
2. 8 g fat (1.5 g saturated)
3. 12 g protein
4. 490 mg sodium
5. 56 g carb
6. 3 g fiber

Cauliflower Fried Rice

Prep time: 20 minutes, cook time: 20 minutes, servings: 2

Ingredients

- 1/3 large head cauliflower
- 2 tbsp vegetable oil
- 1 orange pepper, cut into thin 1/2" pieces
- 1 scallion, sliced
- 1 2-inch piece ginger, cut into thin matchsticks
- 2 tbsp low-sodium soy sauce
- 2 tsp chili garlic paste
- 1 tsp honey
- 2 large eggs
- 1/2 cup frozen peas, thawed
- 1/2 cup frozen edamame, thawed

Directions

1. Cut the cauliflower into florets, discarding the tough inner core and leaves. Working in batches, transfer the cauliflower to the bowl of a food processor. Pulse until the cauliflower resembles rice, about 15 seconds (be careful not to over-process or cauliflower will get mushy). You should have about 4 cups of cauliflower.
2. Heat 1 tablespoon oil in a large cast-iron skillet over medium-high heat. Add the pepper, the white parts of the scallion, and the ginger. Cook for about 2-3 minutes stirring often. Add the cauliflower, toss to combine and cook, covered, stirring once, for 5 minutes.
3. Meanwhile, in a large mixing bowl, whisk together the soy sauce, chili garlic paste, and honey. In another small bowl, lightly beat the eggs. Push the cauliflower mixture to one side of the skillet, add the remaining 1 tablespoon oil, then the eggs, scrambling until cooked, 2 minutes.
4. Remove skillet from heat and fold in the eggs, sauce, peas, and edamame. Serve with thinly sliced scallion greens and enjoy.

Nutrition facts per serving

- 251 calories
- 13.5 g fat (2 g saturated)
- 186 mg cholesterol
- 449 mg sodium
- 15 g protein
- 20 g carb
- 6 g fiber

Lasagna-Stuffed Spaghetti Squash

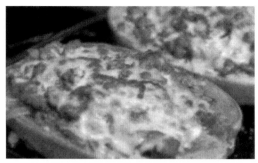

Prep time: 20 minutes, cook time: 20 minutes, servings: 2

Ingredients

- 1 small spaghetti squash (about 1 -1/2 pound)
- 1/2 cup unsalted cottage cheese
- 1/4 cup grated Romano cheese
- Salt and pepper, to taste
- 4 oz frozen broccoli florets, thawed, squeezed of excess moisture and chopped
- 1/4 cup low-sodium marinara or tomato sauce
- 3 oz part-skim mozzarella, grated
- Green salad, for serving

Directions

1. Using a large knife, cut the spaghetti squash in half lengthwise. Use a spoon to scrape out and discard the seeds.
2. Place all 2 squash halves, cut side down, on a large piece of parchment paper in the microwave. Cook on high power until just tender, 8-10 minutes.
3. Meanwhile, heat broiler and lower the rack to the middle position of the oven. In a bowl, combine the cottage cheese, Romano cheese and season with black pepper to taste. Fold in the broccoli.
4. Season the squash halves with salt and pepper, then use a fork to scrape up most of the squash strands, leaving them in the squash. Divide the cheese mixture among the squash and top with the sauce, then the mozzarella. Broil until the filling is

heated through and the top is golden brown, 2 to 3 minutes. Serve with a green salad, if desired.

Nutrition facts per serving

- 217 calories
- 8,5 g fat (4,5 g saturated)
- 26 mg cholesterol
- 476 mg sodium

Quinoa Bowl with Red Pepper, Green Beans, and Red Onion

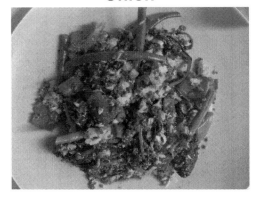

Prep time: 10 minutes, cook time: 15 minutes, servings: 2

Ingredients

- 1/2 cup uncooked quinoa
- 1/4 tsp salt
- 1/4 tsp pepper
- 1 jarred roasted red pepper
- 2 oz green beans
- 1 small red onion, chopped
- 1 tbsp olive oil
- 2 tsp red wine vinegar

Directions

1. Place quinoa in a medium saucepan and pour with 2 cups water. Bring to a boil, add some salt, then reduce heat and simmer, covered, until all the liquid has absorbed, nearly 10 minutes.
2. While cooking, in a large bowl, whisk together oil and vinegar, season with salt and pepper, stir to combine. Add red peppers, beans, and onion and toss to combine. Add the prepared quinoa mix evenly. Serve.

Slow Cooker Honey Mustard Pork with Spinach Rice

Prep time: 10 minutes, cook time: 2-3 hours, servings: 2

Ingredients

- 1/2 pound pork tenderloin
- 1 medium Granny Smith apple
- 1/2 medium onion
- 1 tbsp flour
- 3 medium carrots, cut into 2" pieces
- 2 tbsp Dijon mustard
- 2 tbsp honey
- 1 tbsp low-sodium soy sauce
- 2 sprigs fresh thyme
- 1/2 cup long-grain white rice
- 1 cup baby spinach

Directions

1. Using a food processor, coarsely grate the apple and onion. Add to a slow cooker. Toss with the flour, then the carrots.
2. In a medium mixing bowl, combine the mustard, honey, and soy sauce. Cut the pork in half, place in the slow cooker, then coat with the sauce and nestle it among the vegetables. Scatter the thyme sprigs on top. Cover and cook on high until the pork is cooked through and the carrots are just tender, 2-2 1/2 hours.
3. 25 minutes before the pork is finished, cook the rice according to package directions.
4. Transfer the pork to a cutting board and thinly slice. Discard the thyme from the slow cooker, then fold in the spinach. Serve the pork and vegetables over the rice, spooning the extra apple, onion and juices over the top. Serve and enjoy.

Nutrition facts per serving

- 444 calories
- 5 g fat (1,5 g saturated)
- 74 mg cholesterol

- 471 mg sodium
- 30 g protein
- 67 g carbs
- 5 g fiber

Pasta with Walnut Pesto and Peas

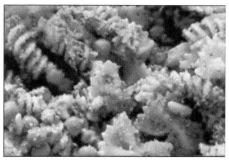

Prep time: 10 minutes, cook time: 20 minutes, servings: 2

Ingredients

- 6 oz. farfalle or other short pasta
- 2 tbsp olive oil
- 1 small onion, chopped
- A pinch of salt
- 1/2 lemon
- 1/4 cup walnuts, toasted
- 1 clove garlic, minced
- 1/4 cup grated Parmesan, plus more for serving
- 1 cup frozen peas, thawed
- 1/4 cup dry white wine

Directions

1. Cook the pasta according to package directions. Reserve 1/2 cup cooking liquid, drain the pasta and return it to the pot.
2. Meanwhile, heat 1 tablespoon oil in a large skillet over medium heat. Add the onion, season with salt and ground black pepper to taste and cook, covered, stirring occasionally, until tender, 6 to 8 minutes.
3. While the onions are cooking, using a vegetable peeler, remove 3 strips of zest from the lemon. Thinly slice the zest; add it to a food processor along with the walnuts and garlic and pulse until finely chopped. Add the Parmesan, 1/4 cup peas, remaining 2 tablespoons oil, and 1/2 teaspoon each salt and pepper and purée until smooth.

4. Add the wine to the onions and simmer for 2 minutes. Add the remaining cup peas and cook, tossing, until heated through. Toss the pasta with the walnut pesto (adding some of the reserved cooking liquid if the pasta seems dry). Add the onion mixture and toss to combine. Serve with a squeeze of lemon juice and additional Parmesan, if desired.

Nutrition facts per serving

- 558 calories
- 21 g fat (3,5 g saturated)
- 4 mg cholesterol
- 458 mg sodium
- 18 g protein
- 77 g carbs
- 6 g fiber

Potsticker Stir-Fry

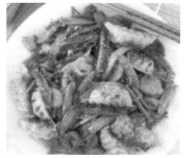

Prep time: 10 minutes, cook time: 25 minutes, servings: 2

Ingredients

- 2 tbsp olive oil
- 8 frozen vegetable potstickers
- 2 tbsp low-sodium soy sauce
- 1 tsp honey
- 2 scallions, sliced
- 1 small red chili, sliced
- 1 clove garlic, minced
- 1 tbsp finely grated fresh ginger
- 6 oz sugar snap peas
- 1 small carrot, cut into matchsticks
- 1 small yellow pepper, cut into 1/2" slices

Directions

1. Heat 1 tablespoon oil in a large skillet over medium heat. Add the potstickers and cook until lightly browned on all sides, 3-5 minutes. Sprinkle with 2 tbsp water to the skillet, cover and cook until the water has evaporated and the potstickers are cooked through, 1 to 2 minutes; transfer to a plate.
2. In a medium-sized bowl, whisk together the soy sauce and honey.
3. Heat the remaining tablespoon oil and add the scallions, chili, garlic, and ginger and cook, stirring, for 1 minute. Add the snap peas, carrot, and pepper and toss to combine. Cover and cook, shaking the pan occasionally, for 2 minutes. Uncover and

continue cooking, shaking the pan occasionally, until the vegetables are tender.

4. Add the soy sauce mixture and toss to combine. Return the pot stickers to the pan and toss with the vegetables.

Nutrition facts per serving

- 270 calories
- 12 g fat (2 g saturated)
- 0 mg cholesterol
- 617 mg sodium
- 10 g protein
- 33 g carbs
- 5 g fiber

Black Bean and Avocado Salsa

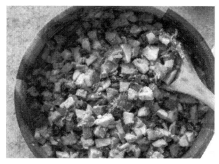

Prep time: 10 minutes, cook time: 15 minutes, servings: 2

Ingredients

- 1/2 can black beans
- 1 garlic clove, minced
- 1 jalapeño pepper
- 1 small onion, chopped
- Salt and pepper to taste
- 2 scallions
- 2 tbsp. fresh lime juice
- 1 tbsp. olive oil
- 1 medium-sized avocado
- 1 tsp dried cilantro

Directions

1. In a large bowl, combine chopped jalapeño, garlic, onion, and season with salt and pepper.
2. Add beans, scallions, lime juice, and oil and toss to combine. Fold in the avocado and cilantro.
3. Serve and enjoy!

Pineapple and Black Bean Fajitas

Prep time: 10 minutes, cook time: 25 minutes, servings: 2

Ingredients

- 1 (15-oz) can black beans, rinsed
- 1 tbsp finely chopped chipotles in adobo
- 1/4 small pineapple, cored and cut into thin 1/2" pieces
- 2 small red peppers, sliced
- 1 small red onion, thinly sliced
- 4 small corn tortillas, warmed
- Fresh cilantro, for serving
- Sour cream, for serving

Directions

1. Heat oven to 425 F or an outdoor grill to medium-high. Tear off four 12" squares of foil and arrange on two baking sheets.
2. Toss together the beans and chipotles, then divide among the pieces of foil. Top with the pineapple, peppers and onion. Cover with another piece of foil and fold each edge up and over three times. Roast or grill (covered) for 15 minutes.
3. Transfer each packet to a plate. Using scissors or a knife, cut an "X" in the center and fold back the triangles. Spoon the mixture into tortillas and top with cilantro and sour cream, if desired.

Nutrition facts per serving

- 229 calories
- 2 g fat (0 g saturated)
- 0 mg cholesterol
- 280 mg sodium
- 9 g protein
- 48 g carbs
- 10 g fiber

Beans and Greens with Lemon-Parmesan Polenta

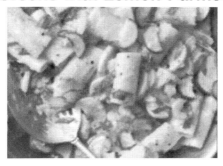

Prep time: 3 minutes, cook time: 20 minutes, servings: 2

Ingredients

- 1/2 lemon
- 1 tbsp olive oil
- 1 small clove garlic, chopped
- 1 tsp fresh thyme leaves
- A pinch red pepper flakes
- 1 small head escarole, trimmed and torn into pieces
- Salt, to taste
- 1/2 (15 oz) can low-sodium white beans, rinsed
- 1 cup instant polenta
- 1 tbsp. unsalted butter
- 1/4 cup Parmesan cheese, grated

Directions

1. Using a vegetable peeler, remove three wide strips of lemon zest; very thinly slice zest.
2. Heat oil in a large Dutch oven on medium. Add garlic, thyme, thinly sliced zest, red pepper flakes and cook, stirring often, until garlic is golden brown, about 2 minutes. Add escarole, in 2 batches if necessary, season with salt and pepper, and cook, stirring occasionally, until escarole is beginning to wilt, about 3 minutes. Reduce heat to medium-low, fold in beans, and cook until escarole is tender and beans are heated through, 2 to 3 minutes more.

3. Meanwhile, cook polenta per package directions. Remove from heat and stir in butter and 1 tablespoon lemon juice, then fold in Parmesan.
4. Serve escarole mixture over polenta.

Nutrition facts per serving

- 335 calories
- 9 g fat (3.5 g saturated)
- 11 g protein
- 530 mg sodium
- 52 g carb
- 10 g fiber

Spaghetti with Grilled Green Beans and Mushrooms

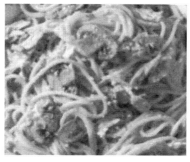

Prep time: 20 minutes, cook time: 20 minutes, servings: 2

Ingredients

- 6 oz whole-wheat spaghetti
- 5 oz cremini mushrooms, trimmed
- 4 oz green beans, trimmed
- 1/2 bunch scallions, trimmed
- 1 1/2 tbsp olive oil
- 1/2 tsp crushed red pepper
- A pinch of salt, to taste
- 2 garlic cloves, minced
- 1 lemons
- Grated Parmesan, for serving

Directions

1. Preheat grill to medium-high. Cook the spaghetti according to package directions.
2. Meanwhile, in a large bowl, toss the mushrooms, green beans, and scallions with the olive oil, crushed red pepper, and 1/2 teaspoon salt. Stir to combine well.
3. Grill the vegetables until just tender for about 4 minutes, then transfer them to a cutting board.
4. Cut the green beans and scallions into 2-inch pieces and place back in the large bowl. Using a garlic press, press the garlic into the bowl, and finely grate the zest the lemons on top. Cut the lemons in half and grill, cut-side down, until charred.

5. Halve the mushrooms and transfer to the bowl along with the spaghetti, squeezing in the juice of the lemons, and tossing to combine. Sprinkle with grated Parmesan, if desired.

Nutrition facts per serving

- 439 calorie
- 9.5 g fat (1.5 g saturated)
- 0 mg cholesterol
- 262 mg sodium
- 17 g protein
- 81 g carbs
- 12 g fiber

Delicious Chickpea & Cauliflower Flatbreads with Avocado Mash

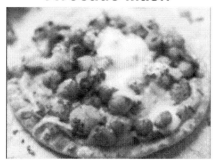

Prep time: 10 minutes, cook time: 25 minutes, servings: 2

Ingredients

- 6 oz cauliflower, cut into florets
- 1 tbsp olive oil
- A pinch of salt
- 1 ripe avocado
- 1 tbsp lemon juice
- 2 flatbreads or pocketless pitas, toasted
- 2 tbsp roasted salted pepitas
- Hot sauce, for serving

Directions

1. Preheat the oven to 420 F. On a large rimmed baking sheet, toss cauliflower with olive oil. Season with salt and pepper and stir to combine. Roast for about 25 minutes.
2. In a mixing bowl mash avocado with lemon juice and a pinch of salt; spread all over flatbreads. Top with roasted cauliflower, chickpeas and pepitas. Serve with drizzle of hot sauce.

Nutritional facts per serving

- 500 calories
- 11 g protein
- 65 g carbs
- 25 g fat (4 g saturated)
- 13g fiber

- 915mg sodium

Heart-Healthy Vegetable Carbonara

Prep time: 10 minutes, cook time: 20 minutes, servings: 2

Ingredients

- 1/2 cup frozen peas
- 1/2 pound spaghetti
- 2 tbsp olive oil
- 1/4 pound asparagus, trimmed and cut into 1/2-inch pieces
- 1 tsp fresh lemon juice
- A pinch of salt, to taste
- 1/4 ground black pepper
- 1 large egg
- 1/4 cup Parmesan, grated
- 1 tsp freshly grated lemon zest
- 8 basil leaves, sliced

Directions

1. Bring a large pot of salted water to a boil. Add peas and cook until just tender, about 2 minutes. Using a slotted spoon, transfer peas to a small bowl. Set aside.
2. Add spaghetti to boiling water and cook just until al dente, about 5-7 minutes. Reserve 3/4 cup pasta water, then drain pasta.
3. While pasta is cooking, heat oil in a 10-inch skillet over medium. Add asparagus and cook, stirring occasionally, until just tender, about 3 minutes. Add peas, sprinkle with salt and cook 2 minutes more. Turn off heat and set pan aside.
4. In a medium-sized bowl, whisk together egg and Parmesan. Add drained pasta and 1/2 cup reserved pasta water and toss to coat well, adding more if necessary.
5. In a mixing bowl, combine asparagus and pea mixture, along with lemon zest, lemon juice, and basil. Season pasta with pepper and additional salt if necessary. Divide among bowls and top with extra Parmesan and basil if desired.

Nutrition facts per serving

- 430 calories

- 10 g fat (3 g saturated)
- 18 g protein
- 450 mg sodium
- 64 g carbs
- 5 g fiber

Heart Healthy Snacks

Grilled Squash Garlic Bread

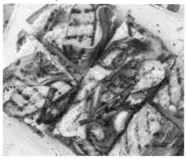

Prep time: 10 minutes, cook time: 20 minutes, servings: 2

Ingredients

- 1 medium-sized zucchini
- 1 summer squash
- 2 tbsp plus 1 tsp olive oil
- Salt and black pepper to taste
- 1/2 bunch scallions
- 1 large ciabatta bread
- 1 large clove garlic
- 1/4 cup ricottta
- 1/4 lemon

Directions

1. Cut zucchini and summer squash lengthwise ¼ inches thick. Brush with 1 tablespoon olive oil, season with salt and pepper, and grill over medium-high until tender, nearly 3 minutes per side.
2. Toss scallions with 1 teaspoon olive oil and grill, turning occasionally, until just tender; transfer to a board and cut into pieces.
3. Split ciabatta bread and toast, then rub each cut side with 1 large clove garlic and brush with 1 tablespoon olive oil.
4. Spread ricotta on each half, then top with zucchini, squash, and scallions. Zest lemon on top and drizzle with 1 tablespoon olive oil.

Nutrition facts per serving

- 325 calories
- 14 g fat (4.5 g saturated)
- 12 g protein
- 530 mg sodium
- 39 g carbs
- 3 g fiber

Spiced Chicken Tacos with Avocado and Pomegranate Salsa

Prep time: 10 minutes, cook time: 10 minutes, servings: 2

Ingredients

- 2 medium boneless, skinless chicken breasts
- 1/2 tsp ground cumin
- 1/2 tsp garlic powder
- 1/4 tsp chipotle chili powder
- A pinch of salt, to taste
- Ground black pepper
- 1 tbsp olive oil
- 4 medium radishes
- 1 scallion
- 1/2 large avocado
- 1/4 cup pomegranate seeds
- 1 tbsp fresh lime juice
- 1/2 cup fresh cilantro leaves
- 4 small flour tortillas
- Sour cream for dressing

Directions

1. Preheat the oven to 425 F. Line a rimmed baking sheet with foil. In a small mixing bowl, combine the cumin, garlic, chili powders, and salt.
2. Heat the oil in a medium skillet over medium heat. Season the chicken with the spice mixture and cook until browned, 2 to 3 minutes per side. Transfer the chicken to the baking sheet and roast until cooked through, 8 to 10 minutes.
3. Meanwhile, in a medium bowl, gently toss together the radishes, scallions, avocado, pomegranate seeds, lime juice, and 1/4 teaspoon each salt and pepper; fold in the cilantro.
4. Slice the chicken into 1/4-inch-thick pieces. Fill the tortillas with the chicken and top with the pomegranate salsa. Serve with sour cream, if desired.

Grilled Fish Tacos

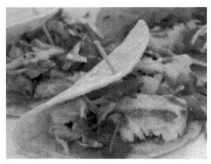

Prep time: 5 minutes, cook time: 15 minutes, servings: 2

Ingredients

- 1 tbsp fresh lime juice
- 1/2 small red onion (finely chopped)
- 1 jalapeño (thinly sliced)
- 1/4 small pineapple (cut into 1/4" pieces)
- 2 medium tomatillos (husks removed and halved)
- 1 pound skinless white fish fillets
- 1/4 cup fresh cilantro leaves
- 4 corn tortillas

Directions

1. In a large mixing bowl, combine lime juice, red onion, jalapeño, pineapple, and season with salt and pepper.
2. Heat grill to medium-high, then grill tomatillos until charred and beginning to soften, 2 to 3 minutes per side.
3. Season skinless white fish fillets with salt and pepper from both sides and grill until lightly charred and opaque throughout, 2 to 4 minutes per side, depending on the fish.
4. Cut the tomatillos into 1/2-inch pieces and fold them into the pineapple mixture along with cilantro.
5. Fill charred corn tortillas with the fish and top with the salsa.

Nutrition facts per serving

- 258 calories
- 3 g fat (0,5 g saturated)
- 54 mg cholesterol

- 204 mg sodium
- 25 g protein
- 33 g carbs
- 3 g fiber

Spinach, Chickpea, and Chicken Pitas

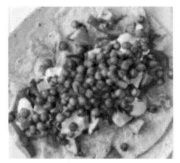

Prep time: 10 minutes, cook time: 20 minutes, servings: 2

Ingredients

- 1/2 small red onion, very thinly sliced
- 2 tbsp red wine vinegar
- 1 tbsp plus 1 tsp extra virgin olive oil
- 2 pieces chicken breasts, boneless and skinless, cut into 3/4" pieces
- 2 cloves garlic, very thinly sliced
- 1 can (15 oz) low-sodium chickpeas, rinsed
- 1 package (10 oz) spinach, thick stems discarded
- 2 pieces pita bread, halved and toasted
- Salt and pepper, to taste
- Greek yogurt, for serving

Directions

1. In a medium-sized bowl, combine the onion, vinegar, and 1 teaspoon oil. Let sit, tossing occasionally, until ready to use.
2. Meanwhile, heat the remaining 1 tablespoon oil in a large nonstick skillet over medium heat. Season the chicken with salt and pepper and cook, tossing twice, until golden brown, 5-6 minutes.
3. Add the garlic and cook, stirring until starting to turn golden brown, 1 to 2 minutes. Add the chickpeas, half the spinach, sprinkle with salt and cook, tossing, until beginning to wilt, about 1 minute. Add the remaining spinach and continue cooking, tossing until just wilted, 1 to 2 minutes; remove from heat.

4. Fill the pitas with the chicken and spinach mixture, top with the onions and drizzle with any vinegar remaining in the bowl. Serve with yogurt, if desired.

Nutrition facts per serving

- 419 calories
- 9,5 g fat (1,5 g saturated)
- 62 mg cholesterol
- 718 mg sodium
- 31 g protein
- 52 g carbs
- 7 g fiber

Spiced Carrot Fritters

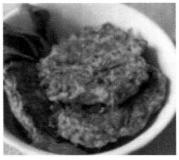

Prep time: 25 minutes, cook time: 30 minutes, servings: 2

Ingredients

- 2 medium eggs
- A pinch of salt
- Black ground pepper
- 2 small carrots
- 1/4 cup Panko breadcrumbs
- 3 scallions, sliced
- 1 red chile, seeded for less heat and thinly sliced
- 1 cup fresh cilantro
- 2 tbsp fresh lime juice
- 3 tbsp olive oil
- 2 oz feta cheese, crumbled
- Green salad, for serving

Directions

1. In a medium-sized mixing bowl, whisk together the eggs and 1/2 teaspoon each salt and pepper.
2. Using a food processor with the large grater attachment, coarsely grate the carrots. Add them to the bowl with the eggs and stir to combine. Cover in breadcrumbs, then in 2 scallions, the chile, and cilantro.
3. In another small bowl, combine the lime juice, 1 tablespoon oil, and remaining scallion.
4. Heat a large cast-iron skillet over medium heat, then sprinkle with 1 tablespoon oil. Drop 6 spoons of the carrot mixture into the skillet and cook until golden brown and crisp, about 3

minutes per side. When ready, transfer to a wire rack. Repeat with the remaining oil and carrot mixture.

5. Gently stir the feta into the lime-scallion mixture. Serve over the carrot fritters and serve with green salad.

Nutrition facts per serving

- 227 calories
- 16 g fat (4.5 g saturated)
- 106 mg cholesterol
- 477 mg sodium
- 7 g protein
- 15 g carb
- 3 g fiber

Turkey Burgers and Slaw with Sweet Potato Chips

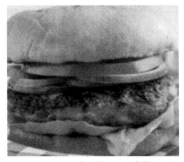

Prep time: 10 minutes, cook time: 25 minutes, servings: 2

Ingredients

Slaw

- 3 tbsp fresh lime juice
- 1 tbsp red wine vinegar
- 1 tbsp honey
- Salt and pepper, to taste
- 4 oz Savoy cabbage, cored and thinly sliced
- 1 small-sized Granny Smith apple, cut into matchsticks
- 1 jalapeño, seeded and thinly sliced
- Sweet Potato Chips and Mayonnaise
- 2 cups sweet potato chips
- 1 tsp smoked paprika
- 1/4 cup mayonnaise
- 1 tbsp Sriracha
- 1 tbsp fresh lemon juice

Burgers

- 1 tbsp chili paste
- 1 tbsp low-sodium soy sauce
- 1 tbsp fresh grated ginger
- 1/2 small onion, finely chopped
- 1/2 pound ground turkey
- 2 tbsp olive oil, for skillet
- 2 buns, split and lightly toasted

Directions

1. Heat oven to 400 F. In a medium mixing bowl, whisk together the lime juice, vinegar, honey, and season with salt and pepper. Mix well. Add the cabbage, apple, and jalapeño and toss to coat. Let sit, tossing occasionally, until ready to serve.
2. Line a large rimmed baking sheet with foil and spread the potato chips in an even layer. Bake just until warm (this releases the oils and helps the spice stick), about 5 minutes. Toss with the paprika.
3. Meanwhile, in a small bowl, whisk together the mayonnaise, Sriracha, and lemon juice; set aside.
4. In a large mixing bowl, whisk together the chili paste, soy sauce, and ginger; stir in the onion, then add ground turkey and mix to combine. Form the mixture into four 3⁄4-inch-thick patties.
5. Heat a grill, or the oil in a large cast-iron skillet, to medium-high heat. Grill or cook the burgers until an instant-read thermometer registers 165 F, 7 to 8 minutes per side on the grill or 4 to 5 minutes per side in the skillet.
6. Spread the buns with a touch of the Sriracha mayonnaise, then top with the burgers and slaw. Serve with the potato chips and remaining mayonnaise.

Nutrition facts per serving

- 735 calories
- 43 g fat (7 g saturated)
- 86 mg cholesterol
- 944 mg sodium
- 29 g protein
- 58 g carbs
- 7 g fiber

Cheesy Artichoke Toasts

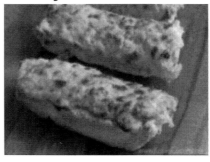

Prep time: 10 minutes, cook time: 15 minutes, servings: 2

Ingredients

- 2 thick slices sourdough bread
- 1/2 (9-ounce) package frozen artichoke hearts, thawed and chopped
- 1 clove garlic, grated
- 2 oz Parmesan cheese, grated
- 1 oz Gruyère cheese, grated
- 1 tbsp sour cream
- 1 tsp finely grated lemon zest plus 1 tablespoon lemon juice
- Salt and freshly ground black pepper, to taste
- 2 tbsp Panko breadcrumbs
- 4 tbsp parsley, chopped
- 1/2 (5-ounce) package baby arugula
- 2 tbsp olive oil

Directions

1. Preheat broiler. Broil bread slices until crisp, for about 2-3 minutes per side. Transfer to a baking sheet and reduce oven temperature to 410 F.
2. In a large bowl, combine artichokes, garlic, Parmesan, Gruyère, sour cream, lemon zest. Season the mixture with salt and pepper to taste and stir to combine. Spoon on toasts and sprinkle with panko.
3. Bake until golden brown and cheese is melted, up to 10 minutes. Sprinkle with chopped parsley, if desired.

4. Meanwhile, in a bowl, toss arugula with oil, lemon juice, and pinch each salt and pepper. Serve with toasts.

Nutrition facts per serving

- 325 calories
- 15.5 g fat (5 g saturated)
- 13 g protein
- 760 mg sodium
- 33 g carbs
- 5 g fiber

Heart Healthy Soups & Stews

Butternut Squash and Turmeric Soup

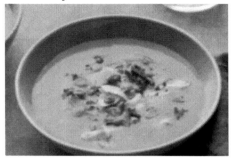

Prep time: 15 minutes, cook time: 35 minutes, servings: 2

Ingredients

- 2 tbsp plus 1 tsp extra virgin olive oil
- 2 small onions, roughly chopped
- 1 tbsp vegetable bouillon base
- About 1 pound butternut squash, peeled (seeds reserved), cut into 1" pieces
- 1 small carrot, cut into 1" pieces
- 2 tsp turmeric
- 2 tsp ground black pepper
- 2 tbsp light coconut milk

Directions

1. Heat 2 tbsp oil in a large Dutch oven over medium heat. Add chopped onion and cook, covered, stirring occasionally, until tender, 6 to 8 minutes.
2. Meanwhile, in a large bowl combine the bouillon base with 6 cups boiling water, stirring to dissolve.
3. Add the squash, carrots, 2 teaspoon turmeric and 1/2 teaspoon pepper to the Dutch oven and cook for 1-2 minutes, stirring well. Add the broth, bring to a boil, then reduce heat and simmer until the vegetables are very tender, 18 to 22 minutes.
4. Meanwhile, heat oven to 375 F. Toss the reserved seeds with 1 tsp of oil, season with additional turmeric and black pepper and roast until golden brown and crispy, for about 10 minutes.

5. Using blender purée the soup. Sprinkle with the toasted seeds and swirl in the coconut milk.

Nutrition facts per serving

- 295 calories
- 15 g fat (5 g saturated)
- 0 mg cholesterol
- 553 mg sodium
- 6 g protein
- 39 g carb
- 7 g fiber

Chickpea and Red Pepper Soup with Quinoa

Prep time: 20 minutes, cook time: 25 minutes, servings: 2

Ingredients

- 1/4 cup uncooked quinoa
- 2 tbsp olive oil
- 1 small onion, chopped
- 1 small carrot, chopped
- 1 stalk celery, chopped
- 2 garlic cloves, minced
- 1 tsp smoked paprika
- A pinch of salt and pepper
- 1 medium yellow bell pepper
- 1 medium red bell pepper
- 1 can low-sodium chickpeas
- 1 cup low-sodium vegetable broth
- 1 tbsp red wine vinegar
- Chopped fresh parsley for garnish

Directions

1. Cook the quinoa according to package directions.
2. While cooking heat the oil in a Dutch oven or large heavy-bottomed pot. Add the onion, carrot, and celery and cook, covered, stirring occasionally, for 6 minutes.
3. Then, add garlic, paprika, season with salt and pepper and cook, stirring, for 1 minute. Add bell peppers and cook for another 5 minutes.
4. Add the chickpeas, broth, and 1 cup water and bring to a boil. Reduce heat and simmer until the vegetables are tender, 5 to 8 minutes. Stir in the vinegar and cooked quinoa. Serve topped with parsley, if desired.

Low-Calories Minestrone Soup

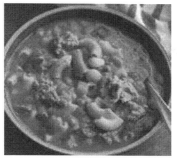

Prep time: 5 minutes, cook time: 25 minutes, servings: 2

Ingredients

- 2 tbsp olive oil
- 1 stalks celery, chopped
- 1 leeks (white and light green parts only), chopped
- 1 small onion, chopped
- Salt and black pepper, to taste
- 6 oz red potatoes, cut into 1/2-inch pieces
- 4 sprigs fresh thyme
- 1 pound asparagus, trimmed and cut into 1-inch pieces
- 3 oz sugar snap peas, halved
- 1/2 15-oz can white beans, rinsed
- Chopped dill and crusty bread

Directions

1. Preheat oil in a Dutch oven on medium. Add celery, leeks, onion, season with salt and cook, covered, stirring occasionally, until tender, up to 7 minutes.
2. Add cut potatoes, thyme, salt and pepper, 3-4 cups water and bring to a boil, then simmer nearly 10 minutes. Add asparagus and simmer 2 minutes more.
3. Add sugar snap peas and beans and simmer until vegetables are tender, for 3-5 minutes more.
4. Discard thyme sprigs. Sprinkle soup with dill and serve with bread and enjoy.

Nutrition facts per serving

- 290 calories
- 7.5 g fat (1 g saturated)
- 12 g protein
- 535 mg sodium
- 46 g carb

14 g fiber

Corn and Potato Chowder in a Slow Cooker

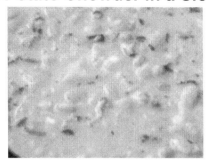

Prep time: 20 minutes, cook time: nearly 5 hours, servings: 2

Ingredients

- 6 oz red potatoes, cut into 3/4-inch pieces
- 1 small onion, chopped
- 1/2 bulb fennel, cut into 1/4-inch pieces, plus fronds for serving
- 1/2 cup frozen corn
- 2 cloves garlic, chopped
- 2 oz cured chorizo, cut into 1/4-inch pieces
- 1 tbsp all-purpose flour
- Salt and freshly ground black pepper to taste
- 2 cup low-sodium chicken broth
- 3 sprigs fresh thyme
- 1/4 cup half-and-half

Directions

1. In a 5 to 6 quart slow cooker, toss the potatoes, onion, fennel, corn, garlic, and half the chorizo with the flour and season with salt and pepper. Stir to combine.
2. Stir in the chicken broth and thyme and cook, covered, until the potatoes are tender, 5 to 6 hours on low or 3 1/2 to 4 1/2 hours on high.
3. Ten minutes before serving, cook the remaining chorizo in a skillet over medium-high heat, tossing occasionally until browned and crisp, 3 minutes.
4. Discard the thyme sprigs from the chowder, and then stir in the half-and-half. Sprinkle the crispy chorizo and fennel fronds over the top, if desired.

Nutrition facts per serving

- 311 calories
- 12 g fat (4 g saturated)
- 26 mg cholesterol
- 600 mg sodium
- 15 g protein
- 37 g carb
- 4 g fiber

Another Way Heart Healthy Minestrone Soup

Prep time: 10 minutes, cook time: 20 minutes, servings: 2

Ingredients

- 1/2 pound asparagus, trimmed and cut into 1-inch pieces
- 1/2 can white beans, rinsed
- 2 tbsp olive oil
- 1 stalk celery, chopped
- 1 leek (white and light green parts only), finely chopped
- 1 small onion, chopped
- 2 medium-sized potatoes, cut in 1/2-inch pieces
- 3 sprigs fresh thyme
- 3 oz. sugar snap peas, halved
- Some freshly chopped dill for serving
- A pinch of salt and pepper to taste

Directions

1. Heat oil in a Dutch oven on medium. Add celery, leeks, onion, season with salt and pepper and cook, covered, stirring occasionally, until tender.
2. Add potatoes, thyme, and 6 cups water and bring to a boil, then simmer 8 minutes. Add asparagus and simmer 2 minutes.
3. Add sugar snap peas and beans and simmer until vegetables are just tender, 3 to 4 minutes more. Discard thyme sprigs. Sprinkle soup with dill and serve.

Slow Cooker Curried Butternut Squash Stew

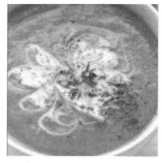

Prep time: 20 minutes, cook time: nearly 6 hours, servings: 2

Ingredients

- 1/2 15-ounce can light coconut milk
- 1 1/2 tbsp vegetable bouillon base
- 1 tbsp curry powder
- 1 tbsp turmeric
- 1/2 tsp cardamom
- 3 tbsp grated fresh ginger
- Salt to taste
- 1 1/2 cup yellow split peas, rinsed
- 1/2 15-ounce can diced tomatoes
- 1 pound butternut squash, peeled and cut into 1/2-inch pieces
- 1 small onion, chopped
- 4 tbsp cup olive oil
- 2 tbsp lemon juice plus 1 teaspoon zest (from 1 lemon)
- 1 large scallion, sliced
- Rice and plain yogurt, for serving

Directions

1. In a 6-quart slow cooker bowl, whisk together coconut milk, vegetable bouillon base, curry powder, turmeric, cardamom, 1 tablespoon grated ginger, 4 cups water, and 1 teaspoon salt. Mix well.
2. Add split peas, tomatoes (and their juices), cut butternut squash, and onion and mix to combine. Secure the lid and cook, covered, until most of the liquid has been absorbed and lentils are tender, 6 to 7 hours on low or 41/2 to 5 hours on high.

70

3. Meanwhile, make lemon-scallion drizzle. In a medium-sized bowl, whisk together olive oil, lemon juice and zest, scallions, remaining 2 tablespoon grated ginger, and 1⁄4 teaspoon salt.
4. Serve the stew with rice and a dollop of yogurt. Drizzle with lemon-scallion drizzle.

Nutrition facts per serving

- 582 calories
- 21.5 g fat (8 g saturated)
- 0 mg cholesterol
- 1,552 mg sodium
- 21 g protein
- 80 g carb
- 24 g fiber

Slow Cooker Pork with Spinach Rice

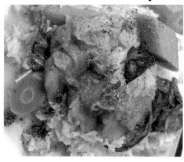

Prep time: 15 minutes, cook time: 2 hours, servings: 2

Ingredients

- 1/2 pound pork tenderloin
- 1/2 cup long-grain white rice
- 1 small green apple
- 1 small onion
- 1 tbsp flour
- 1 cup baby spinach
- 2 large carrots (about 1/2 pound), cut into 2-inch pieces
- 2 tbsp Dijon mustard
- 2 tbsp honey
- 1 tbsp low-sodium soy sauce
- 4 sprigs fresh thyme, plus extra leaves for serving
- Salt and pepper to taste

Directions

1. Chop apple and onion and add to a slow cooker bowl. Toss with the flour and then add carrots.
2. In another mixing bowl combine mustard, honey and soy sauce. Cut the pork into 2 pieces and place to a slow cooker. Pour with the mustard mixture and mix to combine. Sprinkle with salt and pepper and add some thyme on top.
3. Secure the lid and cook until carrots are tender, about 2 hours.
4. Meanwhile, cook rice according the package directions.
5. Open the lid and discard the thyme. Transfer the meat to the cutting board and slice it. Add baby spinach to the slow cooker

and stir to combine well. Serve sliced pork with rice and veggies, sprinkle with some fresh dill or cilantro if desired.

Heart Healthy Salads

Heart Healthy Pear & Walnut Salad

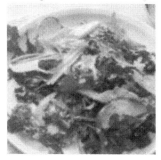

Prep time: 10 minutes, cook time: 10 minutes, servings: 2

Ingredients

- 1/2 cup walnuts
- 1 tsp apple pie spice
- 2 tbsp lemon juice
- 2 tbsp olive oil
- 1/2 tsp salt
- 1/4 tsp pepper
- 2 stalks celery
- 1 large Bartlett pear
- 1 bulb fennel
- 1 scallion, sliced
- 2 small bunches arugula, stems trimmed

Directions

1. On a baking sheet, toss ½ cup walnuts with 1 tsp apple pie spice and roast at 400 F for about 10 minutes or until fragrant. Then, roughly chop.
2. Whisk together 2 tbsp each lemon juice and olive oil, ½ tsp salt, and ¼ tsp pepper in a large mixing bowl. Stir to combine well.
3. Add 2 stalks celery, 1 Bartlett pear, 1 bulb fennel, and 1 scallion (all thinly sliced) and toss to combine.

4. Just before serving, toss 2 small bunches arugula (thick stems discarded) with pear mixture and serve with spiced nuts.

Nutrition facts per serving

- 200 calories
- 15.5 g fat (2 g saturated)
- 4 g protein
- 295 mg sodium
- 15 g carb
- 5 g fiber

Delicious Sugar Snap Peas and Radish Salad

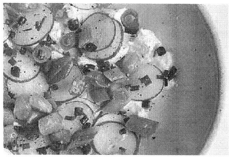

Prep time: 10 minutes. cook time: 10 minutes, servings: 2

Ingredients

- 1 pound sugar snap peas
- 12 small radishes
- 1/2 medium ripe avocado
- 2 tbsp. apple-cider vinegar
- 1 tbsp. fresh lemon juice
- 1/2 tsp. Dijon mustard
- 1/2 tsp. salt
- 1/2 tsp. Freshly ground pepper
- 1/4 tsp. ground coriander
- 3 tbsp olive oil

Directions

1. In a large bowl, combine sugar snap peas and radishes. Set aside.
2. In a blender or the bowl of a food processor, combine avocado, vinegar, lemon juice, mustard, salt, pepper, and coriander. Gradually add oil, blending until mixture is a smooth purée. If needed add couple tbsp water.
3. Toss salad with dressing to coat and serve immediately.

Leek and Lemon Linguine

Prep time: 5 minutes, cook time: 25 minutes, servings: 2

Ingredients

- 6 oz. whole-wheat linguine or spaghetti
- 2 tbsp olive oil
- 2 cloves garlic, thinly sliced or minced
- 1 medium leek, white and light green parts cut into half-moons
- 1/2 lemon
- 1 cup frozen peas
- 1/4 cup fresh flat-leaf parsley, roughly chopped
- 1/4 cup Parmesan, finely grated
- A pinch of salt
- Black pepper

Directions

1. Bring a large pot of water to a boil and season with salt. Cook the pasta according to package directions; reserve 2 cups cooking liquid, then drain.
2. Meanwhile, in a large deep skillet heat the oil over medium heat. Add the garlic and cook, stirring, until lightly golden brown, for about 1-2 minutes. When ready, using a slotted spoon, transfer to a paper towel-lined plate. Add the leeks to the pan, season with 1/2 teaspoon salt and cook, stirring occasionally until tender, 6-8 minutes.
3. Meanwhile, using a vegetable peeler, remove 4 strips of lemon zest. thinly slice the zest on a diagonal. Squeeze 2 tablespoons juice into a small bowl and set aside.
4. Add the peas, whole parsley leaves and lemon zest to the skillet along with 1 cup of reserved cooking liquid and simmer gently for 2 minutes. Add the drained pasta, Parmesan, reserved garlic and 1/2 teaspoon pepper tossing to combine, then toss with the lemon juice, adding extra pasta water if the pasta seems dry. Sprinkle with the chopped parsley and serve with extra Parmesan, if necessary.

Nutrition facts per serving

- 510 calories
- 14 g fat (3 g saturated)
- 9 mg cholesterol
- 518 mg sodium
- 20 g protein
- 84 g carbs
- 12 g fiber

Chicken Fajita Salad with Lime-Cilantro Vinaigrette

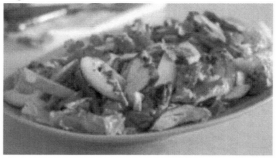

Prep time: 10 minutes, cook time: 25 minutes, servings: 2

Ingredients

- 2 8-oz chicken breasts, boneless and skinless
- 2 small peppers (orange and yellow), quartered lengthwise
- 1 jalapeño, halved lengthwise
- 1 small onion, sliced into 1/2" thick rounds
- 3 tbsp. plus 1 tsp. olive oil
- 1/2 avocado
- 1 lime
- 1 tsp honey
- 1 packed cups cilantro (trimmed, including thin stems)
- 1 small heart romaine, leaves separated, halved if large
- Kosher salt and pepper

Directions

1. Heat grill to medium-high.
2. Season the chicken with salt and pepper from both sides. In a large mixing bowl, toss the peppers and onion with 1 tablespoon oil and season with salt, to taste Cut the avocado in half, remove the pit, and gently rub with 1 teaspoon oil.
3. Grill the chicken until cooked through, 7 to 8 minutes per side; transfer to a cutting board. Grill the vegetables until just tender, 4 to 6 minutes per side, transferring them to a cutting board as they are done. Grill the avocado, cut side down, until charred, 1 to 2 minutes.
4. Slice the peppers, separate the onions into rings, and dice the avocado. Let the chicken rest until ready to serve, then slice.

5. Finely grate the zest of 1 lime into a blender. Squeeze in 6 tablespoon lime juice. Add the honey, cilantro, and remaining 2 tablespoon oil and purée until smooth.
6. Toss the romaine with 1/4 cup of the dressing and top with the sliced peppers, onions, avocado, and chicken. Serve with the remaining dressing.

Nutrition facts per serving

- 358 calories
- 21,5 g fat (3,5 g saturated)
- 63 mg cholesterol
- 313 mg sodium
- 26 g protein
- 17 g carbs
- 6 g fiber

Avocados with Creamy Crab Salad

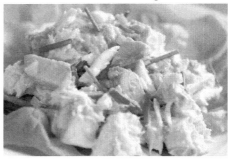

Prep time: 3 minutes, cook time: 5 minutes, servings: 2

Ingredients

- 3 firm ripped avocados
- 1 tbsp grated lemon zest
- 4 tbsp fresh lemon juice
- 1 pound lump crab meat
- 1/4 cup radishes, diced
- 4 tbsp light mayonnaise
- 1 tsp dried basil

Directions

1. Cut 2 avocados in half. Chop remaining avocado in 1/2-inch dice. Sprinkle 2 tablespoons of the lemon juice over halved and diced avocados.
2. In large bowl combine diced avocado, lemon zest, the remaining 2 tablespoons lemon juice, crab meat, radishes, mayonnaise, and basil, tossing lightly.
3. Spoon mixture into the cut halves of avocado.
4. Serve with grilled or toasted pita bread if desired.

Ratatouille Salad

Prep time: 20 minutes, cook time: 30 minutes, servings: 2

Ingredients

- 1 large red pepper, quartered
- 1 small eggplant, sliced into 1/4" rounds
- 1 medium zucchini, sliced lengthwise into 1/4" strips
- 1 small summer squash, sliced lengthwise into 1/4" strips
- 1 lb Campari or plum tomatoes, halved
- 2 1/2 tbsp olive oil
- A pinch of salt, to taste
- Freshly ground black pepper, to taste
- 2 tbsp red wine vinegar
- 1/4 cup fresh basil, leaves torn
- 4 cup baby arugula
- 2 large thick slices sourdough or country bread
- 1 clove garlic, halved
- 4 oz fresh mozzarella, crumbled

Directions

1. Heat your grill to medium-high.
2. In a medium-sized bowl, mix the vegetables with 1 1/2 tablespoons oil and 1/2 teaspoon each salt and pepper. Stir to combine well. Grill until lightly charred and tender, 3 to 4 minutes per side for the pepper, eggplant, zucchini, and squash, and 1 to 2 minutes on the cut side only for the tomatoes. Transfer the eggplant and tomatoes back to the bowl and the rest of the vegetables to a cutting board.
3. Slice the peppers, zucchini, and squash and add to another bowl. Gently toss with the vinegar, basil, and arugula.
4. Brush the bread slices with remaining tablespoon oil and grill until lightly toasted, 1 to 2 minutes per side, then rub both sides with the cut side of the garlic clove.
5. Cut each slice of bread in half and transfer to plates. Spoon the salad and any juices over the bread, then top with the mozzarella.

Nutrition facts per serving

- 309 calories
- 17 g fat (5.5 g saturated)
- 7 mg cholesterol
- 452 mg sodium
- 12 g protein
- 30 g carb
- 6 g fiber

Heart Healthy Chicken Recipes

Roasted Chicken and Garlic Potatoes with Red Pepper

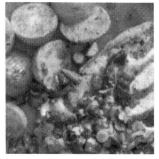

Prep time: 20 minutes, cook time: 40 minutes, servings: 2

Ingredients

- 1 pound potatoes, halved
- 4 tbsp olive oil
- 2 cloves garlic (2 cloves smashed)
- 1/2 tsp salt
- 1/4 tsp ground black pepper
- 2 chicken breasts, boneless and skinless
- 1/2 cup roasted red peppers, drained and cut into ¼-inch pieces
- 1 scallions, chopped
- 1/4 cup roasted almonds, chopped
- 3 tbsp vinegar
- 2 tbsp chopped flat-leaf parsley

Directions

1. Preheat oven to 425°F. On a large rimmed baking sheet, toss potatoes with 2 Tbsp oil. Mince 2 cloves garlic over top, sprinkle with 1/4 tsp salt, and toss to combine. Roast 15 minutes.
2. Meanwhile, heat a large skillet on medium-high. Season chicken with salt and pepper. Add 1 tbsp oil to skillet, then add chicken and cook until browned, about 4 minutes for the each side.
3. Turn chicken over, add smashed garlic to skillet, and cook 1 minute more. Transfer skillet to oven along with potatoes and roast until chicken is cooked through and potatoes are golden

brown and tender, 6 to 8 minutes more; transfer chicken and garlic to a cutting board.

4. Meanwhile, in medium-sized mixing bowl, combine peppers, almonds, scallions, vinegar, remaining tbsp oil. Season with salt and pepper to taste. Chop smashed garlic, add to pepper mixture along with parsley, and mix to combine. Serve with chicken and potatoes. Enjoy!

Nutrition facts per serving

- 520 calories
- 23.5 g fat (3.5 g saturated)
- 40 g protein
- 590 mg sodium
- 38 g carb
- 6 g fiber

Slow Cooker Chicken Marbella for Two

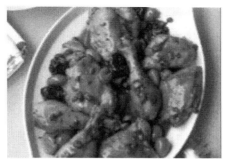

Prep time: 15 minutes, cook time: nearly 5-6 hours, servings: 2

Ingredients

- 1/4 cup dry white wine
- 1 tbsp brown sugar
- 1 tsp dried oregano
- 3 tbsp red wine vinegar
- Salt and pepper
- 4 cloves garlic, minced
- 1 tbsp capers
- 1/4 c prunes
- 1/4 cup pitted green olives
- 2 small chicken legs, split (4 drumsticks, 4 thighs)
- 1/4 cup fresh flat-leaf parsley
- 1/2 cup long-grain white rice

Directions

1. In a 5-6-qt slow cooker, whisk together wine, brown sugar, oregano, 2 tablespoons of the vinegar, and season with salt and black pepper, to taste. Add minced garlic, capers, prunes and olives and mix to combine.
2. Add the chicken, nestling it among the olives and prunes. Cover the lid and cook until the meat is tender and cooked through, on low for 5 to 6 hours or on high for 3 to 4 hours; gently stir in the remaining tablespoon vinegar and parsley.
3. Thirty minutes before serving, cook the rice according to package directions. Serve the chicken, prunes, olives and cooking liquid over the rice.

Nutrition facts per serving

- 480 calories
- 9 g fat (2 g saturated)
- 36 g protein
- 490 mg sodium
- 64 g cards
- 3 g fiber

Chicken Fillets Marinated in Yogurt

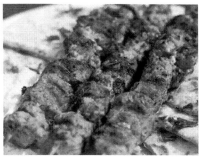

Prep time: 30 minutes, cook time: 30 minutes, servings: 2

Ingredients

- 1 pound chicken breasts, boneless and skinless, cubed into 2-inch pieces
- 1/2 cup non-fat yogurt
- 2 garlic cloves, minced
- 1 tbsp grated ginger
- 1/2 tsp curry powder
- 1 tbsp lemon zest, grated
- 2 tbsp lemon juice
- 1 large bell pepper cut into 2-inch pieces
- 1 tbsp oil
- Salt and pepper to taste

Directions

1. In a large mixing bowl, combine the yogurt, garlic, ginger, curry powder, lemon zest, 2 tablespoons lemon juice. Season with salt and pepper and stir to combine. Add chicken cubes and set aside for 15 minutes.
2. Preheat your grill to medium-high. Thread the chicken and peppers onto skewers. Lightly oil the grill and cook the kebabs, turning couple times, until cooked through, 8 to 10 minutes.
3. Serve with rice, couscous or vegetables.

Sesame Chicken and Chili Lime Slaw

Prep time: 10 minutes, cook time: 15 minutes, servings: 2

Ingredients

- 2 large egg whites
- 2 5-oz chicken breasts, boneless and skinless
- 4 tbsp sesame seeds
- 1 tbsp olive oil
- 4 tbsp lime juice
- 1 tbsp grated fresh ginger
- 1 tsp. honey
- 1 small red chili, thinly sliced
- 1/2 small head red cabbage (about 1 1/4 lbs.), cored and finely shredded
- 1 small carrot, peeled and coarsely grated
- 1/4 cup small fresh cilantro leaves
- Salt and pepper, to taste

Directions

1. Heat oven to 425 F. In a large bowl, beat the egg white with ½ tsp salt until combined. Dip the chicken in the egg white, letting any excess drip off, then coat in the sesame seeds; transfer to a plate.
2. Heat a large cast-iron skillet over medium heat. Once hot, add the oil and cook chicken until the side touching the skillet is golden brown, about 5 minutes. Turn the chicken, then transfer the skillet to the oven and roast until the chicken is cooked through, 8-10 minutes.
3. Meanwhile, in a large bowl, whisk together the lime juice, ginger, honey, and ¼ tsp each salt and pepper; stir in the chili. Toss the cabbage and carrots in the dressing to coat, then fold in the cilantro. Serve with the chicken.

Nutrition facts per serving

- 355 calories

- 16 g fat (2,5 g saturated)
- 78 mg cholesterol
- 515 mg sodium
- 36 g protein
- 19 g carbs
- 6 g fiber

Balsamic Chicken with Apple, Lentil, and Spinach Salad

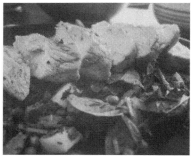

Prep time: 15 minutes, cook time: 20 minutes, servings: 2

Ingredients

- 1 large chicken breast, boneless and skinless
- 1 scallions
- 1 small green apple
- 1 stalk celery
- 1 tbsp fresh lemon juice
- 1/2 can lentils
- 1 cup baby spinach
- 1/4 cup fresh flat-leaf parsley
- 3 tbsp olive oil
- A pinch of salt and pepper to taste
- 2 tbsp balsamic vinegar

Directions

1. Heat 1 tablespoon oil in a large skillet over medium heat. Season the chicken with salt and pepper and cook until golden brown, nearly 6-7 minutes each side. Remove from heat and add the vinegar. Turn the chicken to coat.
2. While cooking, in a large bowl, place scallions, apple, celery, lemon juice, 1 tablespoon oil, season with salt and pepper. Fold in the lentils, spinach and parsley (if desired) and serve with the chicken.

Savory "Fried" Chicken

Prep time: 20 minutes, cook time: 30 minutes, servings: 2

Ingredients

- 4 small chicken drumsticks (about 1 pound), skinless
- 1/4 cup buttermilk
- 2 tsp non-salt blackening seasoning
- 1/4 tsp salt
- 2 cup cornflakes
- 1 tbsp olive oil
- 1/4 cup fresh flat-leaf parsley, chopped

Directions

1. Preheat the oven to 375 F. Line a rimmed baking sheet with nonstick foil.
2. In a small shallow bowl, combine the buttermilk, blackening seasoning and season with salt, to taste. Mix well.
3. Finely crush the cornflakes and transfer to another large bowl. Toss with the oil, then add chopped parsley.
4. Dip the chicken in the buttermilk, letting any excess drip off, then coat in the cornflakes, pressing gently to help them adhere. Transfer to the prepared baking sheet.
5. Cook until the chicken is golden brown and cooked through, 30 to 35 minutes.

Nutrition facts per serving

- 244 calories
- 8.5 g fat (2 g saturated)
- 95 mg cholesterol
- 619 mg sodium
- 28 g protein
- 14 g carb
- 1 g fiber

Sweet and Spicy Chicken Stir-Fry

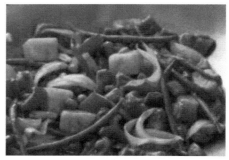

Prep time: 10 minutes, cook time: 15 minutes, servings: 2

Ingredients

- 1 pound chicken breasts, boneless and skinless
- 1/2 cup brown rice
- 1/2 cup apricot preserves
- 2 tbsp cider vinegar
- 1 tbsp grated fresh ginger
- 1/4 tsp crushed red pepper flakes
- 3 tsp canola oil
- 2 medium carrots
- 1/2 pound snow peas

Directions

1. Cook the rice according to package directions.
2. Meanwhile, in a small bowl, combine the apricot preserves, vinegar, ginger, red pepper flakes and 1 Tbsp water; set aside.
3. Heat the oil in a large skillet over medium-high heat. In batches, cook the chicken until golden brown, 1 to 2 minutes per side; transfer to a plate.
4. Add the carrots, snow peas and remaining tsp oil and cook, tossing, for 2 minutes. Return the chicken to the skillet, add the apricot mixture, and cook until the chicken is cooked through and the vegetables are just tender, 2 to 3 minutes more. Serve over the rice.

Baked Chicken Cutlets with Pineapple Rice

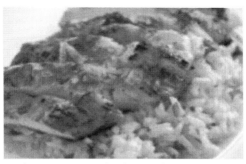

Prep time: 7 minutes, cook time: 15 minutes, servings: 2

Ingredients

- 1/2 cup long-grain white rice
- 1/4 c. reduced-sodium soy sauce
- 1 tbsp rice vinegar
- 1 tbsp grated fresh ginger
- 4 small chicken cutlets (about 1 pound)
- 1 cup Panko breadcrumbs
- 1 1/2 tbsp canola oil
- 1 small red chili, thinly sliced
- 1/4 small pineapple, cored and cut into thin 1/2" pieces
- 1/2 cup fresh cilantro leaves

Directions

1. Preheat oven to 450 F. Line a baking sheet with nonstick foil. Cook rice according to package instructions.
2. Meanwhile, in medium mixing bowl, combine the soy sauce, vinegar and ginger; transfer half to a large bowl and toss with the chicken.
3. Place panko in a shallow bowl and toss with oil. Coat each cutlet in panko and transfer to prepared baking sheet. Bake until golden brown and cooked through, 10-12 minutes.
4. Fluff rice with a fork and toss with chili, pineapple, and cilantro. Serve with chicken cutlets and reserved sauce.

Nutrition facts per serving

- 529 calories

- 9 g fat (1,5 g saturated)
- 78 mg cholesterol
- 689 vg sodium
- 37 g protein
- 72 g carbs
- 3 g fiber

Delicious Chicken Stir-Fry with Rice

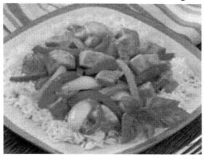

Prep time: 15 minutes, cook time: 30 minutes, servings: 2

Ingredients

- 1/2 pound chicken breasts, boneless and skinless
- 1/2 cup brown rice
- 1/4 cup apricot preserves
- 1 tbsp vinegar
- 1 tsp ginger, grated
- A pinch of red pepper flakes
- 3 tbsp olive oil
- 1 medium-sized carrot
- 1/4 pound snow peas

Directions

1. Cook the rice according to package directions.
2. While rice is cooking, in a medium mixing bowl combine apricots, vinegar, grated ginger, pepper flacks and some water. Set aside.
3. Cut lengthwise chicken breasts. Preheat the skillet oven medium-high heat and roast chicken until golden brown, for about 3-5 minutes per side. Transfer to a plate.
4. Add chopped carrots, snow peas and some oil to the skillet and cook for 2-3 minutes, stirring occasionally. Return the chicken fillets to the skillet, pour over the apricot mixture and cook for another 3-4 minutes until vegetables become tender.
5. Serve with rice and enjoy!

Yogurt-Marinated Chicken Kebabs

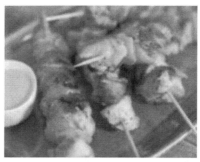

Prep time: 10 minutes, cook time: 20 minutes, servings: 2

Ingredients

- 1/2 cup plain yogurt
- 2 cloves garlic, finely chopped
- 1 (1-inch) piece ginger, peeled and grated
- 1/2 tsp curry powder
- 1/4 tsp ground cloves
- 1 tbsp grated lemon zest
- 3 tbsp lemon juice
- 1 pound chicken breasts, boneless and skinless, cut into 1 1/2 inch pieces
- 1/2 cup couscous
- 1 red pepper, cut into 1 1/2 inch pieces
- 1 tbsp vegetable oil
- 1/4 c fresh mint, roughly chopped
- 2 oz crumbled feta cheese (about 1/2 cup)
- Salt and black pepper, to taste

Directions

1. In a medium mixing bowl, combine the yogurt, garlic, ginger, curry powder, ground cloves, lemon zest, 2 tablespoons lemon juice. Season with salt and pepper and stir to combine well. Add the chicken and let sit for 15 minutes.
2. Place the couscous in a large bowl, add 1 1/4 cups hot water, cover and let sit for 15 minutes.

3. Heat grill to medium-high. Thread the chicken and peppers onto skewers. Lightly oil the grill and cook the kebabs, turning occasionally, until cooked through, 8 to 10 minutes.
4. Fluff the couscous with a fork and fold in the oil, the remaining tablespoon lemon juice, then the mint, and feta. Serve with the kebabs.

Nutrition facts per serving

- 401 calories
- 10 g fat (3 g saturated)
- 77 mg cholesterol
- 455 mg sodium
- 33 g protein
- 42 g carbs
- 4 g fiber

Heart Healthy Chicken Pitas
Prep time: 10 minutes, cook time: 15 minutes, servings:2

Ingredients

- 2 large plum tomatoes
- 1/4 small sweet onion
- 1 tbsp olive oil
- Salt and black pepper to taste
- 2 cups cooked, shredded white meat chicken
- 1/2 cup roughly chopped fresh flat-leaf parsley
- 2 piece pita bread
- 1 container hummus
- 1/4 head romaine lettuce
- 1/4 cup roughly chopped fresh mint leaves
- 1 small lemon

Directions

1. In a medium-sized mixing bowl, toss together the tomatoes, onion, oil, and 1/4 teaspoon each salt and pepper. Add the chicken and parsley and toss to combine.
2. Split the pitas to make 4 rounds. Spread each with hummus, then top with the lettuce and mint and squeeze the juice of half the lemon wedges on top.
3. Spoon the chicken salad on top of the lettuce. Serve with the remaining lemon wedges.

Heart-Healthy Turkey Meatballs

Prep time: 10 minutes, cook time: 15 minutes, servings: 2

Ingredients

- 1/2 pound lean ground white meat turkey
- 1 large egg white
- 4 scallions, 2 finely chopped and 2 thinly sliced
- 1 tbsp chopped fresh dill
- 1 tsp cumin
- 1/2 tsp coriander
- A pinch of salt
- Freshly ground black pepper, to taste
- 1 small lemon, halved
- 2 peppers (1 orange and 1 red), quartered, then thinly sliced crosswise
- 1 jalapeño, seeded and thinly sliced
- 1/2 cup small grape or cherry tomatoes, halved
- 1 tbsp olive oil
- 1/2 cup low-fat plain Greek yogurt
- 2 thin pitas

Directions

1. Heat broiler and line a large rimmed baking sheet with nonstick foil.
2. In a large bowl, combine the turkey, egg white, chopped scallions, dill, cumin, coriander, and season with salt and pepper. Shape the mixture into 10 small patties and place on the prepared sheet. Broil until just cooked through, 4 to 5 minutes. Squeeze the juice of half a lemon over the top.
3. In another large bowl, squeeze the juice of the remaining lemon half. Add the peppers, jalapeño, tomatoes, oil, sliced scallion, and salt and pepper. Toss to combine.
4. Spread the yogurt on the pitas, top with the burgers and spoon the pepper relish over the top.

Nutrition facts per serving

- 424 calories
- 13,5 g fat (3 g saturated)
- 78 mg cholesterol
- 658 mg sodium
- 33 g protein
- 43 g carbs
- 4 g fiber

Heart-Healthy Turkey Lettuce Cups

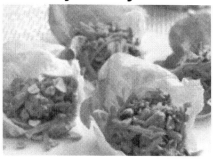

Prep time: 5 minutes, cook time: 15 minutes, servings: 2

Ingredients

Turkey Lettuce Cups

- 1 tbsp canola oil
- 1 pound lean white ground turkey
- 2 cloves garlic, chopped
- 1 jalapeño, chopped
- 1 tbsp ginger, grated
- 1 tbsp low-sodium soy sauce
- 2 tbsp lime juice
- Some water, if it seems dry
- 1 scallions, thinly sliced
- 4 butter lettuce leaves

Cilantro sauce

- 1 chopped jalapeño (seeds off)
- 2 tbsp fresh lime juice
- 1/4 cup plain yogurt
- 1 cup cilantro, freshly chopped
- 1/4 tsp ground cumin

Directions

1. Preheat canola oil in a large cast-iron skillet on medium-high. Add ground turkey and cook, breaking it up with a spoon until golden brown and crispy. Cook for about 8 minutes. Add garlic,

jalapeño, and freshly grated ginger and cook, tossing, for 1 minute.

2. Remove from heat, add low-sodium soy sauce, lime juice, and up to 1/4 cup water (if it seems dry).
3. Sprinkle with scallions. Spoon into butter lettuce leaves and serve with cilantro sauce.

Cilantro sauce

4. Transfer all sauce ingredients to the blender, and purée until very smooth.

Nutrition facts per serving

- 250 calories
- 6 g fat (1.5 g saturated)
- 43 g protein
- 285 mg sodium
- 5 g carb
- 1 g fiber

Seafood and Fish Heart Healthy Meals

Crunchy Tortilla Fish Sticks with Purple Cabbage Slaw

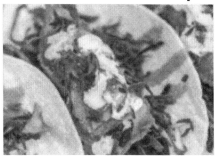

Prep time: 15 minutes, cook time: 20 minutes, servings: 2

Ingredients

- 1 navel orange
- 4 tbsp fresh lime juice
- 1 tsp sugar
- A pinch of salt, to taste
- Freshly ground black pepper to taste
- 1/4 cup sour cream
- 1 small carrot, grated
- 1 small red onion, chopped
- 1/2 pound red cabbage, cored and shredded
- 1 pound tilapia fillets
- 2 cups tortilla chips, crushed
- 1/4 cup fresh cilantro, chopped

Directions

1. Preheat oven to 420 F. Finely grate 1 tsp zest from orange into a large bowl, then squeeze in juice (about 1/4 cup). Add in lime juice, sugar. Season with salt and pepper and whisk in sour cream. Stir to combine. Transfer 1/2 cup mixture to a shallow bowl and set aside. Add carrots, onion, and cabbage to the large bowl and let sit, tossing occasionally, 15 minutes.
2. Meanwhile, line a rimmed baking sheet with foil. Cut tilapia into large chunks. Dip fish in reserved sour cream mixture and then in crushed chips, pressing gently to help them adhere.

3. Transfer fish chunks to the baking sheet and cook until light golden brown and opaque throughout, nearly 10 minutes. Fold cilantro into slaw and serve with fish.

Nutrition facts per serving

- 410 calories
- 13.5 g fat (4.5 g saturated)
- 39 g protein
- 710 mg sodium
- 36 g carb
- 4 g fiber

Cod with Crispy Green Beans

Prep time: 10 minutes, cook time: 20 minutes, servings: 2

Ingredients

- 1/2 pound green beans
- 2 tbsp olive oil
- 1/4 cup Parmesan, grated
- Salt, to taste
- A pinch of freshly ground black pepper
- 1 pound skinless cod, cut into 4 pieces
- 2 tbsp basil pesto

Directions

1. Heat oven to 425 F. On a large rimmed baking sheet, toss the beans with 1 tablespoon oil, then add grated Parmesan, and season with salt and pepper, to taste. Roast until light golden brown, 10-12 minutes.
2. Meanwhile, heat the remaining tablespoon oil in a large skillet over medium-high heat. Season the cod with salt and pepper and cook until golden brown and opaque throughout, about 3 minutes per side; transfer to plates.
3. Spoon the pesto over the cod and serve with the beans.

Nutrition facts per serving

- 242 calories
- 11 g fat (2 g saturated)
- 61 mg cholesterol
- 481 mg sodium
- 27 g protein
- 10 g carbs

Pesto Salmon Burgers with Asparagus and Tomato Salad

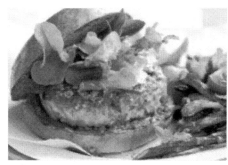

Prep time: 20 minutes, cook time: 15 minutes, servings: 2

Ingredients

- 1/2 pound asparagus, trimmed and cut into 2-inch pieces
- 3 tbsp olive oil
- 1 pound salmon fillet, skinless, cut into 1-inch pieces
- 2 scallions, thinly sliced
- 2 rolls, split and toasted
- 2 tbsp prepared pesto
- 1 cup mixed greens
- 1/2 pound small tomatoes (such as cocktail, Campari, or plum), quartered

Directions

1. Preheat broiler. On a large rimmed baking sheet, toss the asparagus with 1 tablespoon oil, salt and pepper. Broil until just tender, up to 4-5 minutes.
2. Meanwhile, place the salmon in a food processor and pulse couple minutes just until coarsely chopped (it should still be somewhat chunky). Add half the scallions, season with salt and pepper and pulse 2 times to combine. Form the mixture into four 3/4-inch thick patties.
3. Heat 1 tablespoon oil in a large non stick skillet over medium heat and cook the patties, turning once (do not press or flatten), until opaque throughout, 2 to 3 minutes per side. Transfer to rolls and top with pesto and greens.

4. In a large bowl, toss together the tomatoes, asparagus, remaining scallions, remaining tablespoon of oil and 1/4 teaspoon each salt and pepper; fold in the mint. Serve with the salmon burger.

Nutrition facts per serving

- 512 calories
- 13 g fat (4 g saturated)
- 71 mg cholesterol
- 589 mg sodium
- 39 g protein
- 39 g carbs
- 6 g fiber

Scallops with Lemon and Capers

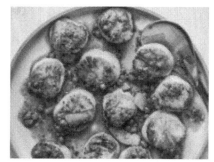

Prep time: 5 minutes, cook time: 10 minutes, servings: 2

Ingredients

- 1 cup low-sodium chicken broth
- 1 tbsp capers
- 1 1/2 tsp cornstarch
- 1 clove garlic
- 1 tsp. grated lemon zest
- 2 tbsp. fresh lemon juice
- Salt and black pepper, to taste
- 3 tsp unsalted butter
- 1 pound sea scallops
- 2 tbsp fresh flat-leaf parsley

Directions

1. In medium mixing bowl, whisk together the broth, capers, cornstarch, garlic, lemon zest and juice, season with salt and pepper, and mix well until the cornstarch dissolves.
2. In large skillet, melt 2 tsp of the butter over medium-high heat. When butter just starts to brown, add the scallops and cook until golden and cooked through, 2-3 minutes per side. Transfer the scallops to a plate.
3. Add the broth mixture to the skillet and bring to a boil. Simmer until slightly thickened, about 1 minute. Remove from heat and stir in the remaining 1 tsp butter and the parsley. Spoon over the scallops.

Tuscan Bass with Squash and Beans

Prep time: 10 minutes, cook time: 15 minutes, servings: 2

Ingredients

- 2 (3 oz) striped bass
- 1 tbsp olive oil
- 1/2 cup sliced onion
- 12 oz zucchini and/or yellow squash
- 2 cloves garlic. minced
- 1/2 can cannellini beans
- 1/2 can tomato sauce
- 1/2 cup water
- 1 tsp chopped fresh rosemary
- 1/4 tsp black pepper

Directions

1. Heat 1 1/2 tsp of the oil in a large nonstick skillet. Add onion and sauté 3 minutes. Add squash and garlic; sauté 2-3 minutes more until fragrant.
2. Add beans, tomato sauce, water, rosemary and pepper. Stir well and bring to a boil. Reduce heat and place fish on top. Cover and simmer 7 to 8 minutes until fish is just cooked through.
3. On plates, top bean mixture with fish; drizzle with remaining 1 1/2 tsp olive oil.

Delicious Tortilla Fish Sticks with Purple Cabbage Slaw

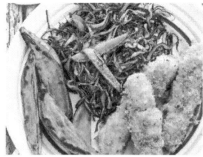

Prep time: 5 minutes, cook time: 25 minutes, servings: 2

Ingredients

- 1 pound tilapia fillets
- 1/2 small red cabbage, cored and finely chopped
- 1 small orange
- 3 tbsp fresh lime juice
- 1 tsp sugar
- 5 tbsp sour cream
- 1 medium-sized carrot, grated
- 1 small red onion, chopped
- 2 cups tortilla chips, crushed
- 1 tsp dried cilantro
- 1/4 tsp salt
- 1/4 tsp pepper

Directions

1. Heat oven to 425°F. Take the large bowl and grate 1 tsp zest from orange into it. Squeeze in juice (about 1/3 cup). Whisk in lime juice, add sugar, salt and pepper to taste, whisk in sour cream.
2. Transfer 1/2 cup mixture to a shallow bowl. Add carrots, onion, and cabbage to the large bowl and let sit.
3. Meanwhile, line a rimmed baking sheet with foil. Cut tilapia into large chunks. Dip fish in reserved sour cream mixture and then in crushed chips, pressing gently to help them adhere.

4. Transfer fish chunks to the baking sheet and cook until light golden brown for about 8-10 minutes. Fold cilantro into slaw and serve with fish.

Shrimp Bowls with Scallion Vinaigrette

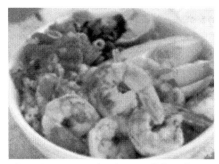

Prep time: 10 minutes, cook time: 20 minutes, servings: 2

Ingredients

- 1 cup quinoa
- 1/2 pound broccoli, cut into small florets
- 2 tbsp olive oil
- Salt and pepper, to taste
- 10 large peeled and deveined shrimp, tails removed
- 1 tbsp rice vinegar
- 1 tbsp finely grated fresh ginger
- 4 oz plum tomatoes, seeds removed and cut into 1/4" pieces
- 2 scallions, thinly sliced
- 1/2 avocado, cut into small pieces

Directions

1. Preheat oven to 425 F. Heat a medium saucepan over medium, add the quinoa, and cook, shaking the pan occasionally, until lightly toasted, 5 minutes. Add 3 cups water and immediately cover (it will sputter). Simmer gently for 10 minutes. Remove from heat, remove lid, cover with a clean towel, and let stand 10 minutes; fluff with a fork.
2. Meanwhile, in a large mixing bowl, toss the broccoli florets with 1 tablespoon oil. Season with salt and pepper and stir to combine. Spread in an even layer over the baking shit and roast

15 minutes. Season the shrimp with a pinch of salt and pepper, toss with the broccoli, and roast until opaque throughout, 6 to 8 minutes.

3. In another mixing bowl, whisk together the vinegar, ginger, and remaining olive oil. Toss with the tomatoes, then fold in the scallions. Divide the quinoa among bowls, then top with the shrimp, the broccoli, and the avocado. Spoon the tomato scallion vinaigrette over the top.

Nutrition facts per serving

- 462 calories
- 19 g fat (2,5 g saturated)
- 58 mg cholesterol
- 457 mg sodium
- 20 g protein
- 57 g carbs
- 12 g fiber

Cod Fillets with Potatoes and Bacon

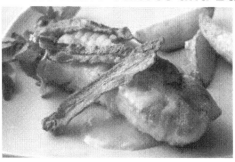

Prep time: 15 minutes, cook time: 15 minutes, servings: 2

Ingredients

- 2 large cod fillets (1 inch thick)
- 2 slices bacon, cut into 1/2-inch pieces
- 1/2 pound small potatoes, halved
- 1 medium red onion cut into 1/2 inch lengthwise
- 1 tbsp. mayonnaise
- 1 tbsp. Dijon mustard
- 5 tbsp panko bread crumbs
- 1 tbsp olive oil
- 1 tbsp Thyme leaves
- Salt and black pepper

Directions

1. Preheat the oven to 450 F. Place potatoes and onions in the center of a baking sheet and place bacon on top. Roast for 10 minutes.
2. While potatoes are cooking, in a medium mixing bowl combine mayonnaise and mustard. In another bowl, combine Panko with oil, then sprinkle with thyme. Season fish with salt and pepper, then spread with mayonnaise mixture and sprinkle with Panko.
3. Remove the baking sheet from the oven and reduce oven temperature to 400 F. Toss potatoes and onion mixture together, then spread in an even layer, arranging potatoes cut side down.
4. Nestle fish pieces among vegetables and roast until fish is tender and lightly golden, for about 10-12 minutes.

Horseradish Salmon Cakes

Prep time: 15 minutes, cook time: 20 minutes, servings: 2

Ingredients

- 2 medium-sized salmon fillets
- 1 tbsp prepared horseradish
- 1 tbsp Dijon mustard
- 5 tbsp Panko bread crumbs
- 2 tbsp olive oil
- 2 tbsp fat-less Greek yogurt
- 1 tbsp fresh lemon juice
- 1 small English cucumber
- A bunch watercress
- A pinch of salt and pepper to taste

Directions

1. In a food processor blend the salmon, horseradish, mustard, salt, and pepper until coarsely chopped. Stir in bread crumbs and form the mixture into 8 patties.
2. Heat 1 tablespoon oil in a large nonstick skillet over medium heat. Cook the patties until brown, 2 minutes per side.
3. In a large bowl, whisk together the yogurt, lemon juice, remaining oil. Season with salt and pepper. Add the cucumbers and toss to coat; fold in the watercress. Serve with the patties.

Sweet and Spicy Glazed Salmon with Delicious Rice

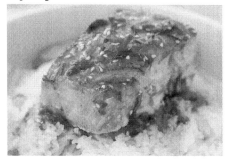

Prep time: 15 minutes, cook time: 25 minutes, servings: 2

Ingredients

- 2 salmon fillets
- 1/2 cup long-grain white rice
- 5 tbsp sliced almonds
- 1 small orange
- 1/4 cup hot pepper jelly
- A pinch of salt and pepper to taste
- Freshly chopped parsley

Directions

1. Heat oven to 390 F. Cook the rice according to package directions.
2. While rice cooking, spread the almonds on a baking sheet and roast until light golden brown, for 5 minutes. Then transfer to a bowl. Heat broiler. Line a broiler-proof rimmed baking sheet with nonstick foil.
3. Squeeze the juice from half an orange into a small bowl and get 2 tablespoons juice. Add the jelly and whisk to combine. Place the salmon on the baking sheet, season with 1/2 teaspoon each salt and pepper, and roast for 5 minutes. Spoon half the jelly mixture over the salmon and broil until the salmon is opaque throughout, 2 to 5 minutes more.
4. Cut remain half of the orange into 1/2-inch pieces. Fold the oranges, almonds, and parsley into the rice. Serve with the salmon and the remaining jelly mixture.

Pistachio Covered Fish

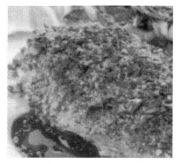

Prep time: 10 minutes, cook time: 15 minutes, servings: 2

Ingredients

- 1/2 cup quinoa
- 2 6-ounce pieces cod or tilapia, skinless
- Salt and ground black pepper, to taste
- 2 tbsp non-fat Greek yogurt
- 1/4 cup whole-wheat Panko
- 1/4 cup unsalted shelled pistachios, chopped
- 2 tbsp olive oil
- 4 cup baby spinach
- 2 tbsp lemon juice

Directions

1. Cook quinoa per package directions.
2. Meanwhile, season fish with salt and pepper, then brush with 1 tablespoon non-fat Greek yogurt.
3. In a large mixing bowl combine whole-wheat Panko and chopped pistachios with 1 tablespoon olive oil. Stir to combine. Sprinkle the mixture over fish, pressing gently to adhere. Bake on a nonstick foil-lined rimmed baking sheet at 375 F until opaque throughout, nearly 12-15 minutes.
4. Fluff quinoa, then add baby spinach, lemon juice, 1 tablespoon oil. Add salt and pepper to taste and toss to combine well, then serve with fish.

Nutrition facts per serving

- 385 calories

- 13.5 g fat (2 g saturated)
- 36 g protein
- 510 mg sodium
- 29 g carb
- 5 g fiber

Shrimp and Garlicky Tomatoes with Kale Couscous

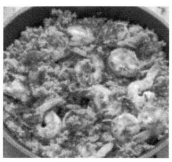

Prep time: 10 minutes, cook time: 20 minutes, servings: 2

Ingredients

- 1 cup couscous
- 1 (5-oz.) package baby kale
- 1/2 pound small cocktail or Campari tomatoes, quartered
- 2 large cloves garlic, minced
- 10 large peeled and deveined shrimp
- 2 tbsp extra-virgin olive oil
- Salt and pepper to taste

Directions

1. Preheat oven to 425 F or an outdoor grill to medium-high. Tear off four 12" squares of foil and arrange on two baking sheets. In a small bowl, combine the couscous with 1/2 cup water.
2. Divide the kale among the pieces of foil. Top with the couscous, then the tomatoes, garlic and shrimp. Drizzle with the oil and sprinkle with salt and pepper.
3. Cover with another piece of foil and fold each edge up and over three times. Roast or grill (covered) for 15 minutes.
4. Transfer each packet to a plate. Using scissors or a knife, cut an "X" in the center and fold back the triangles.

Nutrition facts per serving

- 279 calories
- 8 g fat (1,5 g saturated)
- 44 mg cholesterol
- 469 mg sodium

- 13 g protein
- 40 g carbs
- 5 g fiber

Low Calories Roasted Salmon with Beans & Tomatoes

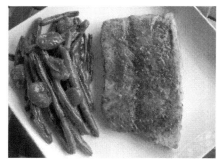

Prep time: 15 minutes, cook time: 20 minutes, servings: 2

Ingredients

- 1 large skinless salmon fillet
- 4 clove garlic
- 1 lb. green beans
- 1 pt. grape tomatoes
- 1/2 c. pitted kalamata olives
- 2 tbsp. olive oil
- kosher salt
- Pepper to taste

Directions

1. Preheat oven to 415 F.
2. In the large bowl mix together the garlic, beans, tomatoes, olives, with 1 tablespoon oil and 1/4 teaspoon pepper. Replace to the baking sheet and roast until the vegetables are tender and beginning to brown.
3. Meanwhile, heat the remaining tablespoon oil in a large skillet over medium heat. Season the salmon with pepper and cook until golden brown and opaque throughout, 4 to 5 minutes per side. Serve with the vegetables.

Tilapia with Rice, Pineapple and Cucumber

Prep time: 15 minutes, cook time: 20 minutes, servings: 2

Ingredients

- 2 medium-sized tilapia fillets
- 1 cup long-grain white rice
- 2 tbsp. fresh lime juice
- 1 tbsp. grated ginger
- 2 tsp. honey
- 2 tbsp. olive oil
- 1 jalapeño pepper, chopped
- 1/2 small pineapple, chopped
- 1 small English cucumber, chopped
- Pepper to taste

Directions

1. Firstly, cook the rice according to package directions.
2. Meanwhile, in a large bowl, whisk together the lime juice, ginger, honey, olive oil and some pepper. Toss with jalapeño, pineapple and cucumber.
3. Heat the remaining tsp oil in a large nonstick skillet over medium heat. Season the tilapia with pepper and cook until golden brown and cooked through, 1 to 3 minutes per side. Serve the fish with the rice and vegetable mixture.

Seared Tilapia with Spiralized Zucchini

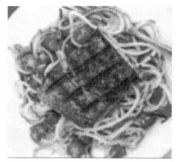

Prep time: 10 minutes, cook time: 15 minutes, servings: 2

Ingredients

- 1 pound zucchini, spiralized
- 3 tbsp olive oil
- 2 small tilapia fillets (nearly 1 pound)
- 1/2 lemon, thinly sliced
- 2 cloves garlic, thinly sliced
- 1 tbsp capers
- 1/4 cup fresh flat-leaf parsley, chopped
- A pinch of salt
- Freshly ground black pepper

Directions

1. Heat oven to 475 F. Line a large rimmed baking sheet with nonstick foil or a reusable baking mat. Using a spiralizer, spiralize the zucchini, or, using a knife, slice zucchini into thin ribbons.
2. Transfer zucchini to prepared baking sheet; toss with 1 tablespoon oil and season with salt & pepper. Roast for 15 minutes. Increase heat to broil and continue to cook until golden brown, 3 to 4 minutes.
3. Meanwhile, heat 1 tablespoon oil in a large cast-iron skillet over medium-high heat. Sprinkle tilapia with salt and pepper and cook until opaque throughout, 2-4 minutes per side. Transfer to plates.
4. Add remaining 1 tablespoon oil to the skillet along with lemon, garlic, and capers and cook, stirring occasionally, until garlic is

golden brown and tender. Toss with parsley, then spoon over tilapia and serve with zucchini.

Nutrition facts per serving

- 289 calories
- 13,5 fat (2,5 saturated)
- 85 mg cholesterol
- 394 mg sodium
- 36 g protein
- 7 g carbs
- 2 g fiber

Roasted Halibut with Orange Salsa
Prep time: 15 minutes, cook time: 15 minutes, servings: 4

Ingredients

Orange Salsa

- 1 medium red onion
- 4 tbsp fresh lemon juice
- 1 navel orange
- 2 pickled jalapeno peppers
- 1/4 cup fresh cilantro

Halibut

1. 2 piece halibut fillet (6 to 8 oz each)
2. Salt and black pepper, to taste
3. Olive oil nonstick spray
4. Directions
5. Prepare Orange Salsa: Toss onion with lemon juice in a medium bowl. Let stand at least 30 minutes, then stir in remaining ingredients.
6. Make Roasted Halibut: Heat oven to 460 F. Line a rimmed baking sheet with foil (for easy cleanup). Place fish on sheet; season with salt and pepper. Coat tops with nonstick cooking spray.
7. Roast 10 minutes or until cooked through. Serve with Orange Salsa.

Fish Chowder Sheet Pan Bake

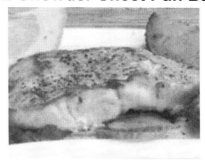

Prep time: 15 minutes, cook time: 15 minutes, servings: 2

Ingredients

- 1/2 pound small yellow potatoes, halved
- 1 small red onion, cut into 1⁄2-inch-thick wedges
- 2 slices bacon, cut into 1⁄2-inch pieces
- 1 tbsp mayonnaise
- 1 tbsp Dijon mustard
- 1 tsp lemon zest, grated
- 1/4 cup Panko breadcrumbs
- 1 tbsp olive oil
- 1 tbsp Thyme leaves
- 4 6-ounce pieces cod fillet (at least 1-inch thick)
- Black pepper and salt to taste

Directions

1. Preheat oven to 450 F. Pile potatoes and onions in the center of a rimmed baking sheet and place bacon on top. Roast for 10 minutes.
2. Meanwhile, in a medium-sized mixing bowl, combine mayonnaise, mustard, and lemon zest.
3. In another bowl, combine panko with oil, then add in thyme. Season fish with salt and pepper, then spread with mayonnaise mixture and sprinkle with panko.
4. Remove the baking sheet from the oven and reduce oven temperature to 425 F. Toss potatoes and onion mixture together, then spread in an even layer, arranging potatoes cut side down.

5. Nestle fish pieces among vegetables and roast until fish is opaque throughout and potatoes are golden brown and tender, nearly 15 minutes.
6. Serve and enjoy.

Nutrition facts per serving

- 412 calories
- 18 g fat (5 g saturated)
- 84 mg cholesterol
- 435 mg sodium
- 33 g protein
- 28 g carb
- 3 g fiber

Conclusion

Thank you for downloading this book!

You will soon make the best dishes ever and you will impress everyone around you with your home cooked meals!

Just trust us! Get your hands on an air fryer and on this useful air fryer recipes collection and start your new cooking experience!

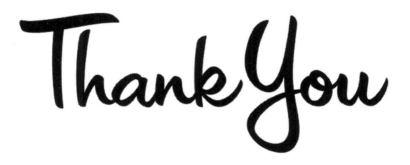

Made in United States
Orlando, FL
28 February 2025

59019241R00070